Pot Farm

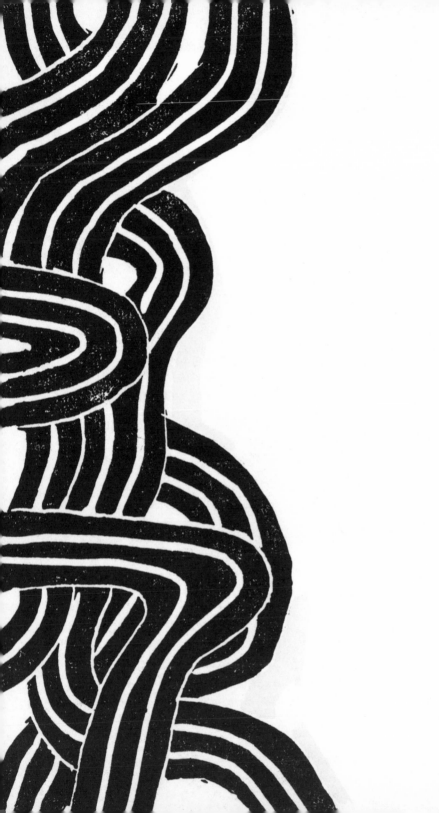

Pot
Farm

Matthew Gavin Frank

University of Nebraska Press
Lincoln and London

Library of Congress
Cataloging-in-Publication Data
  Frank, Matthew Gavin.
Pot farm / Matthew Gavin Frank.
    p. cm.   ISBN 978-0-8032-3784-1
(paperback: alkaline paper)
    1. Marijuana industry—California.
2. Marijuana—Therapeutic use.
    3. Cannabis. 4. Frank, Matthew
Gavin. 5. Agricultural laborers—
    California—Anecdotes. I. Title.
HD9019.M382U64 2012
    331.7'633790979415—dc23
2011031406

Set in Electra by Bob Reitz.
Designed by Nathan Putens.

For Hud Goliath and PSG

One

I WOULD SAY: At dusk, the crops' silhouettes held to the sky like herons cemented into the earth, leaves flapping feebly in the Northern California wind, unable to lift themselves from the forthcoming hands of the Morning Pickers, and the watchful green eyes of Lady Wanda—I would say that, but I was likely stoned. It's just as likely that the crops didn't look like herons at all, there was no wind, and it might not have even been dusk. It could have been morning. It could have been afternoon. Having worked on a medical marijuana farm, filling six notebooks with scribblings of varying degrees of sense, and engaging along the way in the attendant and standard subcultural vices, I have made of myself an unreliable narrator.

Indeed, much of my memory of the experience exists somewhere between the hazy and the disturbingly vivid—it is the stuff of fever dream and emotion, and drugs, and hangovers, and hard physical labor. The pot farm, and that stage in our lives, still has a tenuous feel, an uncertain connection to reality. But that's exactly what the place and that time were: tenuous. I have, by default, forgotten certain things, and am deliberately going to leave others out, like how, on our drive out to California, my wife and I stopped along I-80 to sleep in a small town outside Lincoln, Nebraska, one day after a tornado had destroyed much of the region. I am going to leave out the detail of the giant yellow Super 8 Motel sign that lay crushed in the middle of Main Street.

I am going to try not to dwell on the details of our lives up to this point: How we moved into my parents' house after my mom was diagnosed with cancer, and how, because my father still works six days a week, and they maintain three large dogs, my wife and I became responsible, for just over a year, for the animals' feeding, walking, watering, and shit removal. How we slept on an air mattress in the bedroom I grew up in (I will certainly leave out any discussion about how weird it was to have sex there, in that room where I discovered masturbation and fantasized about the "popular" girls while listening to a cassette of Bon Jovi's *Slippery When Wet*, because everybody writes about that), and always, before falling asleep, cried too much, laughed too much, talked too much, were too fucking silent.

I'm also not going to talk about how that stint drove us to do something deliberately foreign and "off the grid," the way people do when they realize, but are fleeing from, the awareness that they may have just shed their youth, or whatever it was that allowed them carefreedom. How we quietly said goodbye to ourselves, packed up the car, and took off West, thinking, without saying it, that we could somehow have a hand in jump-starting a new phase in our lives. Some people have children, or shave their heads. We took off for the pot farm—not because we're a marijuana-crazy couple or anything, but because it sounded like the experience could spark . . . well . . . something.

Given the nature of the pot farm and the people who work there, I am changing names as well as not talking about certain things. Unreliable. I am Binjamin Wilkomirski, and James Frey, and Helen Demidenko, and Wanda Koolmatrie. I am waiting to be crucified on *Oprah*, then sign a seven-figure deal.

So: I was likely stoned, and let's say it was dusk, and let's say the crops looked like some kind of water bird. My wife and I strolled the first few rows before the communal dinner, our shoes picking up soil as we moved. I do remember that: the place was soily, though *soily*'s not a word (and *soil-rich* sounds too "green," and *soiled* sounds like a dirty diaper). Unreliable.

I must admit: I'm a little neurotic about engaging the whole "mom-with-cancer" thing. Books about such events seem ubiquitous these days, and I hope you don't think that this is one of *those* stories. I do have to warn you, though: It's likely to come up again, but only to further the main thread—the pot farm thread—and to provide a dramatic (and truthful!) backdrop, such as in "a passionate love story set against the backdrop of the post-revolution '30s and '40s Mexico" (Jonathan Holland, review of *Tear This Heart Out, Variety*, December 19, 2008).

So: In Mendocino County, summer confuses itself with fall; fall with winter. Likewise, the seemingly dissonant landscapes commingle—rocky headland shore, redwood forest, and wine country overlap, yielding an environmental cassoulet that somehow works together. You can fact-check that. I'm pretty sure I'm right.

The crops average just over six feet tall, looking down on my wife and me as if concerned parents, hands on their hips, braced to praise or punish. Behind us, the sun wounds the sky, and scores of tents from the Residents' Camp whip like sails—another would-be moveable species held in place with cement shoes, or stakes, or the bodies of the weary crew.

As you may have noticed, I'm switching to present tense. That's my choice, I feel, even though this happened in the past. I'm hoping it lends this tale some of the same paranoiac urgency I felt while living it. If you care about that sort of thing, then . . .

We can hear the tinkling chorus of four acoustic guitars making their way through a mocking, overwrought rendition of Journey's "Don't Stop Believin'." (Here, I probably rolled my eyes and mocked a dry heave—my usual response to Journey—though secretly I was also choking down an uncool reflex to hoist my right fist into the air. Maybe I should have felt more comfortable being myself around my wife; after all, we'd been married for five years at that point. What was wrong with me?)

As the moon asserts itself, the guitars suddenly go quiet, one of the singing voices missing the cue, left stranded without music: *Hold on to that feeee-lay-eee-aayng!* I am quietly jealous of the picking crew. They seem so at ease making asses out of themselves, which is to say, being human. I feel I can learn something from them.

A dull orange cloud of Durban Poison smoke hangs over the Residents' Camp tonight. This exotic strain of medical marijuana was only this morning the bane of our existence, as the Pickers were asked to trim even more quickly and carefully than usual.

"We have three times the requests for D.P. than any other," Lady Wanda told us this morning. "More than Northern Lights, more than Trainwreck."

That Lady Wanda allows some favored Pickers to sample such an in-demand product speaks to her benevolence. As Johanna and I watch the sky drain itself of light, the Residents' Camp seems to yawn as one. Some crew members take naps before dinner, some take walks, some stretch and meditate at the evening yoga class in Lady Wanda's cavernous basement, some sit alone and smoke their paycheck, enjoying the crop.

I nod to Hector, one of the Treetop Snipers, who is stationed fifty feet up a south-leaning redwood, even though I know full well that since he is on duty, he would never nod back. I reach for Johanna's hand. Hers is smooth with oil, mine is still sticky with resin. She's here at Weckman Farm as a resident massage therapist. Her friend Robbi, with whom she grew up in Overkalix, Sweden, is the farm's resident yoga instructor. A thin, well-muscled woman, Robbi is what my robust Jewish grandmother would have called "a little piece of gristle."

Remember, names have been changed. Sometimes, this refers to the names of places. I chose the name *Weckman Farm* because it sounds a little like the farm's real name, though not in the way that you're thinking. Another admission: because I can't see you, I am going to be presumptuous from time to time. Please don't be offended. Also, "Johanna" and "Robbi" are not from Sweden. They are from another non–North American country—one that has seen a bit more unrest in the twentieth and twenty-first centuries.

experience with one of these helicopters—though, of course, I was likely stoned at the time. Sorry.

Each grower is issued a government-certified permit to cultivate a certain number of plants for a fixed number of patients. If an airborne law enforcement official, with binocular aid, suspects that the farm possesses even one more plant than the allowed number, the helicopter will land and, according to Lady Wanda, "All hell will break loose."

In 2005 alone, Lady Wanda warns her crew, employing her favorite slang for the local law enforcement, "Johnny Screw confiscated over a million and a half plants in this county. And stole quite a bit of money as well. They have more guns then we do. We've gotta watch each other's asses."

At this point in her speech, the wind would probably sweep the hem of her flowered housefrock slightly to the left, bestowing on her speech an added emphasis, and presenting the possibility that we might get a glimpse of one of her magnificent thighs. I admit, I now overuse the whole *Johnny Screw* phrase, much to the annoyance of my friends, without citing Lady Wanda as my source. I doubt she's the persecute-for-plagiarism type.

I listen to Lady Wanda, whether she's talking about ass-watching or crate-hauling. Perhaps it's not only her hulk I find intimidating, or the fact that she's managed to domesticate something as wild as the wind, but this is the first time I've ever engaged in employment quite this, well, underhanded. Additionally, rumors circulate among the crew (though nobody claims to have seen it) pertaining to the size of Lady Wanda's gun collection.

Always at her command, I drop my scissors to the soil and carry a crateful of recently trimmed marijuana buds—about six pounds' worth—to the flatbed of a one-seat tractor driven by Charlie the Mechanic. By this time, the sweat ringing the chest of my shirt rivals the expanse of Lady Wanda's sunburn, and I will think of Johanna calmly performing some craniosacral therapy in the air-conditioned comfort of her New Age mausoleum.

A Picker (also known as a Trimmer) is responsible for grooming the marijuana buds with a pair of nail scissors, making them perfect. As with the harvesting of wine grapes and other ingestibles, the pruning of the product is of utmost importance. I reach elbow deep into the plants, the leaves, oils, resin, wayward clippings tattooing my arms with the smell that will stay with me for the season; the smell that permeates my clothes and shoes and tent; the smell that will ruin a chair if I sit down; the smell that will infect a carpet if I stand up.

Everyone on Weckman Farm bears this olfactory burden, though rumors circulate of special soaps and shampoos that almost get rid of it. Of the many rumors saturating Weckman Farm, this is the most often dispelled. It is because of the smell—a jogger bull moose's dirty laundry—that the Pickers are rarely allowed in Lady Wanda's house, save for The Mausoleum. But even her mansion, formidable as a bulwark, is susceptible. Because Johanna sleeps with me, the odor of premature marijuana attaches itself to her and, in turn, Lady Wanda's gothic basement. Pickers talk of growers who, every season, have to replace their furniture.

Reaching into the crop without removing the soon-to-be-smokable bud from the plant, I manicure the stuff, pruning away all rotten segments: marijuana that has grown small tufts of white mold; marijuana that has desiccated too early; the large outer fan leaves that have fallen into brittle dryness. I collect all of these clippings in a crate and carry them to the one-seat tractor. The work itself is hard and monotonous. If the job were legal, these mundane details of my work at the pot farm would be of about as much interest as my summer spent detasseling corn outside Normal, Illinois.

Charlie the Mechanic will not stop staring at me until I successfully deposit the crate on the flatbed, as if he's trying to divine the secret ingredient responsible for the miracle of human locomotion. Every time I set the crate on his tractor (there are many, given that a Picker may opt to work twelve- to fourteen-hour days), Charlie exhales through his nose and speaks his refrain, "That's it, brother."

His voice is trapped in rasp, predicting the tracheotomy he'll certainly have to receive in a decade or so. A two-day-old beard permanently clings to his face like playground sand, and in the early mornings, his hair glows ethereal orange. Never having fully recovered from his tours in Vietnam, Charlie enjoys his Seagrams 7 whiskey a bottle at a time and his Winston cigarettes by the carton.

Rumors spread among the Pickers: some say that Charlie used to be a millionaire oil tycoon and had a fleet of tankers working under his command somewhere in Alaska, but when his wife left him, he went to ruin; some say that when his wife left him, he became an ice cream truck mechanic in Los Angeles. The common denominator is the flight of the wife. Rumor also has it that he occasionally drinks tractor fuel.

Always, at day's end, I tell Johanna what I've heard. This is our favorite predinner ritual.

"You can't believe everything you hear in this place," Johanna tells me as we round one row of pot plants and disappear into another. "Rumor also has it that everyone who works here is a great liar."

By *great*, I hope she means *talented*, but I'm pretty sure she means *big, fat*.

"Maybe they just like to tell a story," I say.

"I'd love to see a list of Lady Wanda's prerequisites," she says, smiling, too tired to laugh at herself.

This is our privacy together, when I can marvel at Johanna's ease with the world. After Chicago, and living for a year in my childhood bedroom, with its autographed photo of Ryne Sandberg and pinup of Alyssa Milano circa *Who's the Boss?* I'm surprised she still can muster it. She's seen so much more of the world than I.

Dusk is slowly giving way to night (or morning to afternoon, afternoon to evening . . . Choose your own adventure). Johanna lets go of my hand and cracks her knuckles. She has given seven hours' worth of massage to the crew today and her hands are hurting her. I've had my hand cuffed into a pair of scissors all day. My hands are hurting me too.

OF COURSE, it took more than Robbi's job offers to bring Johanna and me out here. Should I write about this part in any sort of detail, or would that mean I'd be defying my own vow to keep such things

9

relegated to the realm of "backdrop"? Should I discuss how, in 2006, I found myself living in my parents' house in suburban Chicago for the first time since I was seventeen, this time with Johanna in tow, because of my mom's diagnosis? How, after having lived in Alaska, Italy, Key West, New Mexico, Arizona, and (a failed attempt) Vermont, reentering Buffalo Grove, Illinois, gave me the alcoholic shakes, the only substance that could quell them being the swallowed desire to flee to some distant mountaintop, some beach bungalow, some bomb shelter in which I could grow, with impunity, a wizard's beard beneath which to hide? Oh shit, oh shit. This *is* one of those stories, isn't it? No. No. It's just the establishment of context, right? I can't say *backdrop* and not give the stage curtain a color, right? Right?

Also, I did not change the names of the places I lived. Those are accurate, as is the Buffalo Grove admission, which I'm still a little leery about. I've tried for most of my life to shuck that place, for better or for worse. But hell, I played enough Four Square and Running Bases, and chased enough field mice, and ate enough bad food in that town that I shouldn't fear claiming a small portion of ownership.

Of course, this descent (for Johanna) and redescent (for me) into B.G. at first crept into us like nausea with a remarkable intensity, but then, for the most part, it kept quiet. We were Haleakalā, Mount Edgecumbe, Chato Volcano, and Paulet Island: dormant. On one occasion, at the crest of my mother's therapy, when she was (as she was so often then) sleeping, my father, never one for overt emotion, called me into his bathroom—the same bathroom where, years earlier, I had discovered, in the middle of a stack of *Playboy* magazines kept on the blue-padded laundry hamper (Dad was a subscriber), the December 1984 issue featuring a photo shoot of Karen Velez, images that would not only come to play a crucial role in my later shunning of breast implants but also forever change the way I used and reacted to the word *pendulous*.

Walking quickly, I passed the walls lined with his Howdy Doody and Hopalong Cassidy memorabilia, a display my mother referred to as "his childhood cemetery." In the bathroom, he was standing next to the toilet, hair less curly than it used to be, new totem pole tattoo clinging bright to his left shoulder, staring into the blue wastebasket and shaking his head. Few sights are more pathetic than one's father, nervous beyond reason, standing next to a toilet. Karen Velez and the flightiness by which I had defined myself up to that point were long gone, hopefully commingling in the bottom of the same mid-1980s Dumpster. He gestured at the wastebasket, and I had to slow down. I had to look. Like at a car accident on the highway. Inside the wastebasket, I saw a mound of my mother's brown hair—enough, it seemed, to cover the floor of a barber shop.

"Why do you want to show me this?" I asked him, my throat reacting as it would have to a sliver of black peppercorn.

He snorted softly. He looked confused.

"I think you should share in this," he said.

MANY TIMES, Johanna and I delved into understandable selfishness, lamenting our loss of sanctuary, our rhythms, this wet cloak clinging to our skins, stirring our hearts to a perpetual flutter. Let me rephrase: we were pissed off. Distraught, sure, but *pissed*. We became solitude fetishists. A quiet evening at home, just the two of us, was our autoerotic asphyxiation, a bad late-night action movie our silk stocking. (On bad action movies, see: *Tier One*: anything with Lorenzo Lamas, Brian Bosworth, or Dolph Lundgren [save for *Rocky IV*]; *Tier Two*: anything with Jean-Claude Van Damme, Steven Seagal, or Eric Roberts; *Tier Three*: anything with Schwarzenegger, 1970–88; *Tier Four*: anything with Schwarzenegger, 1989–2003 [with the exception of the—heavy on the quotation marks—"comedies," *Junior*, for example]; *Tier Five*: *Rocky IV*. This list is heavily abridged, the order of tiers inversely proportional to the quantity of alcoholic drinks the viewer has consumed.) Johanna initially dismissed these films as "a load of shit," but by month two, she was just as addicted as I.

Many times we would go for midnight walks to the neighborhood park—the site of my first tornado slide, Little League baseball games, after-school fights; the place where I lost my third tooth, falling from the tire swing; the place where I tried, and succeeded at, eating a woodchip—and sit together on the swing set, sometimes silent, sometimes raging with the urge to flee. Part of me wants to say something about the stars here—a specific constellation, even (Andromeda, my favorite—it has something to do with the sea monster)—but I'm gonna pull back.

We would complain about the way the city lights dampened the night sky, about the ever-listening ears of the neighbors, who were likely descendants of the Original *Yenta*. We would talk about how my mother would surely heal, overusing the words *strong* and *pull through*, and about the many options that lay ahead for us—which looked to me just then, when I closed my eyes, like an endless chain of yellow center highway lines, the lane separators, an even scarier version of the trailer for David Lynch's *Lost Highway*. On that swing set, in that park, we approached each option with equal disinterest. Then, we would go back to the house, undress in my old bedroom, and listen to my parents cough half the night.

ABOUT EIGHT MONTHS LATER, when it looked as if all might turn out well with my mom, my wife and I, lost and insane with the thirst for solitude, and desperate for a measure of cleansing, received Robbi's phone call and decided to take these seasonal jobs. We did this without knowing anything about the Residents' Camp and communal meals, or tent livin', or strange showers that would compel us to wear rubber shoes for fear of contracting all things fungal . . . No, at the time, all we knew was that after an extended diet of midwestern realism, with all of its spiritual bratwurst, moving to California seemed like a chance for a cosmic high-colonic. And Robbi had worked for Lady Wanda before, so we were welcomed with hefty open arms, without much interrogation.

JOHANNA AND I often talk of Chicago during our predinner walks, but we don't tonight. We're too hungry. For the season, Lady Wanda has set up a white canvas carnival tent on the east side of her substantial house, under which three meals a day are served. From the fields, Johanna looks longingly toward the tent's three white peaks as if they were as snow-covered and as insurmountable at the Himalayas. Sometimes, when we're craving meat, they are. After a day of massage, when she's hungry, Johanna can get irrationally poetic about food.

"I hope they shoehorn some lamb into that vegetable mass tonight," she growls.

Meals on Weckman Farm are typically vegetarian but, I must admit, wonderfully prepared. Alex, Emily, and Antonio are the three full-time chefs under Lady Wanda's employ, and just so you don't invest too much in them, I'll tell you now that they will not be major players in this tale. That doesn't mean I can't try to describe them, though. And later on, I may even tell a story or two about them. It depends on how I'm feeling, benevolent or smart-ass, both moods likely disingenuous and forced for the sake of the narrative. But for now, consider Alex and Emily pseudohippie wallpaper, and Antonio a bookshelf-bound and balloon-cheeked bust of Buddha.

Alex and Emily, a married couple in their upper twenties, are culinary school graduates who cut their teeth at a pair of well-known Napa Valley restaurants (he as a sous chef, she as a pastry chef) before finding their way to Weckman Farm. They both wear cat's-eye glasses and beads in their hair and have a flair for breakfasts. This morning we had sea-palm (a local seaweed) quiche with caramelized onion and feta cheese. I tried to like it, and eventually did. Johanna, not the world's biggest fan of ocean-born green stuff, bitched. She decorated the edges of her plate with these lovely little blobs of rejected magnesium.

Antonio, a fifty-year-old man from Veracruz, Mexico, with a robust fifty-year-old paunch, is their sous chef, trained in his mother's restaurant, perfecting such dishes as last night's dinner of enchiladas *suizas* stuffed with roasted mushroom and topped with a tomatillo cream sauce. Though the dish was meatless, we both adored it, and if I remember correctly, Johanna may have clapped once.

Their kitchen is housed in a large blue-roofed shed in Lady Wanda's backyard and includes four ranges, an indoor grill, a chest freezer, a commercial mixer, and a walk-in refrigerator. Johanna speculates that not a single piece of this equipment has ever had the luxury of housing so much as a sliver of lamb.

"I think they fear real protein," she whines, enumerating the oft-repeated list of the exotic meats she enjoyed as a girl growing up in northern Sweden. As always, as if for emphasis, or to subvert the cute and the Christmas-y, she ends her rant with ". . . reindeer!"

I reach for her hand again as we watch Alex, Emily, and Antonio carry plastic-wrapped aluminum food bins from the rear of the house to the picnic benches under the tent. We can hear Antonio grumbling to his *chefs de cuisine*, "If you two don't stop French-kissing when you're supposed to be shucking corn, we're going to be here all night." He rockets a string of what must be the most marvelously obscene Spanish I've ever heard, yanking the plastic wrap from the food. The French-kissing, it must be admitted, happens nightly, though I confess I am occasionally turned on by their public displays of affection. I'm a voyeur. Johanna's fully aware of this. Sue me.

Johanna's hand, which hasn't lost any of its oil from a day of rubbing people, squeezes mine. The aromas of something entirely vegetal float from the tent, infiltrate the breeze, and strike my wife with a leafy disappointment. She sighs the sigh of a woman who is having something green (again!) for dinner; who is living outside for a season in a Coleman Cimarron tent—a Coleman Cimarron amid sixty others in the Residents' Camp. This is not necessarily what we had in mind when chanting the word *sanctuary!* on that swing set back in Chicago.

The Residents' Camp sits like a shantytown village on the opposite end of the property from Lady Wanda's house. Unless the weather turns to rain, or becomes the California version of cold, it's uncommon to see a male crew member wearing a shirt in the Residents' Camp. The few women who make up Lady Wanda's crew have been known, occasionally, to forgo shirts as well. Johanna and I are probably the camp's most *clothed* crew members, though we do feast our eyes on the only meat—some more well-done than others—served here at Weckman.

For a shantytown, amenities abound. Or, if not amenities, an *amenity*. Lady Wanda has constructed a pair of shower sheds in the camp, replete with hot water. They are a pot farm version of clean—which is to say, dirty—and as I said, Johanna and I don our rubber sandals with enthusiasm before we shower. When we first arrived at Weckman Farm, one shed was for the boys, the other for the girls. As the season progressed, things became a bit more co-ed. The curtains are mercifully (again, depending on who you ask) opaque. I'm thinking of Charlie the Mechanic here.

"The world's goin' to shit," Lady Wanda says to the crew after the workday, "but I run my generator on vegetable oil. Enjoy your showers!"

Lady Wanda is a self-proclaimed permaculturalist. I'm not sure that word exists east of the Continental Divide. Pardon my presumptuousness—I just found out that the permaculture movement, whose mission is to construct "human" communities and agricultural setups that resemble the interconnections found in natural ecosystems, began in the 1970s in Australia. The word, in print, tends to keep company with the word *synergy*, and who am I to deprive it of its life partner? Anyhow: praise Wikipedia.

As such a permaculturalist, Lady Wanda has, in Weckman Farm, attempted to create a self-sufficient minisociety that avoids dependence on the many amenities of industry. She sings the financial praises of her role as ecologically inclined businesswoman. Her vegetable oil–powered generator costs her forty cents per gallon.

For a first-time Picker, this self-sufficiency can carry with it the side effects of claustrophobia and stench. Every crew member who arrives by car is instructed to park in an open grassy lot on a spur road off the main gravel drag that leads to Weckman Farm. We have access to our vehicles only in cases of emergency. Often, I picture our reddish Kia Spectra lying dormant, collecting the spoiled smells of our abandoned road snacks. I think we may have ditched half of a turkey salad sandwich beneath the front passenger seat because of Johanna's distaste for the celery brunoise suspended in it. At night, in the tent, I would often think of this sandwich, and bugs, and become anxious and unable to sleep. What can I tell you? I'm a suburban Chicago Jew at base.

Lady Wanda collects lists of her crew's favorite products. She then sends a team of faceless shoppers into the nearest small town (not very near) to gather these items. She labels the resulting paper bags with our names in black magic marker, so we can have access to our Vidal Sassoons, our AquaFreshes, and our SpeedSticks without ever having to leave the premises. If we must send out mail, Lady Wanda collects it and has another faceless messenger truck it to the local (not very local) post office every three days. She even pays our postage. This way, a Picker has very little to do but work; this contained, sustainable world a constant fluctuation between field, food tent, and the Residents' Camp.

The Residents' Camp faces Lady Wanda's mansion as if the two are opposing heads of a medieval table, we workers constantly facing the nighttime, queenly stare of her lit upstairs windows—a royal and intimidating job interview. The atmosphere in the camp is surprisingly courteous, many of the workers putting away their acoustic guitars, djembe drums, and laptop stereos early in the night. After all, many of us are working longer hours than investment bankers.

Johanna and I walk from the pungent crops to the warm mouth of the food tent. The sun has nearly dipped out of sight, only its red scalp hanging on the horizon above the rows. The air is heavy and without definitive season. It can be January or June. It can only be California.

Two

FOR DINNER WE have masa harina corn cakes with herb sauce and a dilled potato salad. Johanna, though dejected at another day of meatlessness, eats voraciously. We all do, really. She and I sit at a rust-painted picnic table with Lance, Crazy Jeff, Gloria, Hector, and Charlie the Mechanic. The field crew eats with hunched shoulders, cramped forearms, aching lower backs. Johanna sits abnormally straight, exhibiting her self-described "perfect body mechanics." We all swat at the flies and mosquitoes as we eat, with the exception of Charlie the Mechanic, who seems oblivious to them. He is oblivious also to the mayonnaise in his beard.

Hector hates the insects the most. A short, stocky man in his forties, he waves wildly at the bugs with both hands, dropping his plastic fork to the ground, retrieving it, and wiping it on his pants, only to begin the process again a moment later.

"These fuckin' bugs eat more than we do," he shouts, frustrated.

"It's the truth, man," Lance says. He speaks in a voice that forever sounds as if it's about to drop off to a decades-long sleep, a voice that sounds *at home*. Or rather: *at hoooooome* . . .

"I'm serious," Hector stresses. "When these fuckers bite us, think about the equivalent. I mean, the food they eat compared to the size of their bodies, and the food we eat compared to the size of ours. It's ridiculous."

Hector's hair, jet black and tightly curled, wobbles as one contained unit as he speaks, swats at his ears, drops his fork, and picks it up again. I have previously encountered such a head of hair only on my late grandmother. I wonder if Hector also spends his Saturdays in the beauty parlor, his hair liberally doused with hairspray and pulled at with a fuchsia teasing comb, or if he, like she, will, after arguing with his offspring for hours about the thermostat setting, silently leave bed in the middle of the night in house slippers and housefrock, and, with hunchback catching the moonlight, raise the temperature a couple degrees while everyone but the grandson is sleeping.

"Yeah," Lance snores, "the equivalent. It's totally unfair."

They both pronounce the word *equivalent* as if they had invented it just moments ago. In their mouths it seems so new, deserving of endless repetition. Of course, they're probably high. Of course, I may be too. Who remembers? When a brain cell falls into the cerebral spinal fluid, and not a single of his compatriots is alive to hear it, does he, in attempting to recall the truth, make a sound?

We make up one table of about twenty. The conversation, for such a crowd, let alone such a crowd of societal rebels, is surprisingly hushed. During our meals, we are not making any large statements, not changing the world or subverting any governments. We are farm laborers, famished and tired, chewing more than we speak. At least at the meal's beginning . . .

Charlie the Mechanic burps demurely, Crazy Jeff laughs to himself, Gloria rotates her head in a circle with an audible crack, and Johanna touches my leg under the table. We can't see the stars beyond the white ceiling of the canvas tent, but out here, tonight, I'd bet they'd be huge.

"Piece-of-shit bugs," Hector says more calmly. "And they're better than us, too." He shoves another wedge of corn cake deep into his mouth.

Hector was born in Chiapas, Mexico, and became an American citizen through, according to him, "some deal with the U.S. Army." His military tattoos cover his thick arms with a sickly vein-green, as if he had some adverse and irreparable reaction to an intravenous medication. I remember that, in our first few days here, he told us stories about how, as a child, he would stalk leopards through the Chiapas jungle, not far from the Guatemala border. I believe him. His military training, and perhaps his résumé as leopard stalker, earned him a place in the treetops. As a Treetop Sniper at Weckman Farm, he serves as an armed guard, keeping watch for trespassers, marijuana poachers, and law enforcement.

This whole sniper thing made Johanna and me, at the beginning of our stay, incredibly uneasy. Johanna particularly has an aversion to guns. One of the reasons she fled her home country was the second attempted carjacking she faced, during which, like the first, she'd had a semiautomatic held to her temple at a stoplight. In response, as during the first, she'd floored the gas pedal, narrowly averting cross-traffic, and run over the guy's foot (and if this doesn't sound much like Sweden to you, give yourself a pat on the frontal lobe). She told me this on our first real date, a breakfast in Key West (where we were both working in restaurants at the time), detailing the image that still plagues her at night of the perpetrator falling over into the street as she watched in the rear view mirror. And I have never—as Paul Hamby, Juneau, Alaska, fireman to whom I served blueberry-pecan pancakes in the Channel Bowl Cafe (where I worked before meeting Johanna), would say it—*discharged a weapon*. But after having dined with Hector a few times, we soon grew accustomed to the notion of "sniper as sweetheart," and other such anomalies unique to Weckman Farm, and this particular line of work.

Hector has an eight-person tent set up at the Residents' Camp, though he rarely stays the night, and when he does, he sleeps in the large tent alone. Sometimes, the picking crew can become indignant regarding Hector's clearance to leave the property, while we are bound to it. On his tent's door, he has stapled a laminated postcard of the Virgen de Guadalupe garlanded with pink carnations.

One night in our tent, before we went to sleep, Johanna asked me, "Do you think he comes from a family of eight? Do you think he gets to sleep imagining the seven other people? Or that the space reminds him of his family?"

Johanna has enough heart for the two of us, though for the sake of tone here, I'm trying to keep mine at bay.

"We don't even know if he has a family," I said.

"We should ask him," she said, fatigue pouring itself into her voice like motor oil.

I love it when her voice sounds like this—it's so tired-sexy—but at the time, I was too sore–hung over to do anything about it.

"If I catch him without his rifle, I'll ask him," I said.

Johanna said nothing. I paused, listening to the night sounds—wind, frogs, insects, the breathing of the crew in their tents.

"I just wonder where he goes at night," I said.

Johanna let out a dull, elongated violin snore.

Now, as Charlie the Mechanic burps at the dinner table again, this time flamboyantly, turning his head to the side and pursing his lips as if sipping from an imaginary, midair water fountain, Johanna touches my leg all the more mightily.

"Shiiiiiit," Lance moans as if the word were four syllables.

"That's it, brother," Charlie rasps.

Lance taps me on the shoulder. When I look up from my paper plate, he says nothing, just sits there nodding with both his hands flat on the table.

Lance is only twenty-four, but this is his fifth season working at Weckman Farm. This makes him a Field Manager or Head Trimmer, both titles referring to the same set of duties: he tells, in his cat-before-a-nap sort of way, the Virgin Pickers (as they're called) how to carefully trim the plants so as not to lose any of the "medicine. This is very, very important." He takes his time with the verys, his shoulder-length blond hair swaying with his voice, calling to the oceanic Southern California rhythms that reportedly encompassed his formative years. This is Lance: slow tide in, slow tide out.

Like any good-looking young guy in a position of authority, Lance is a combination of annoying and enviable. When I listen to him, I have the same reaction I do to a lot of the surfer interviews I've watched: I struggle between wanting to be that surfer and wanting to punch him in the face. Lance probably never knew what it was like to be a nerd, favoring classic rock when all his cool classmates were listening to Bon Jovi's *Slippery When Wet*. In the junior high school gym class locker rooms, he probably never had to pretend to be familiar with lyrics that he had never heard (pleading, "Shot through the *heart*! Shot through the *heart*!") just so Ricky Meyer wouldn't throw wet wads of toilet paper at him and, potentially, bodyslam him onto the changing bench. I heard that Ricky Meyer is now a millionaire. I hate it when bullies become successful.

Lance belongs to one of two factions of the crew who choose to be paid in marijuana. The first is a group who tend not to spend the night at the Residents' Camp, known at the farm as the Patients. The Patients, many of whom work as Pickers, use the marijuana to alleviate the effects of illness. (Despite her agony, I couldn't have possibly convinced my mom to go this route, because "it's illeeegal.")

In the Residents' Camp, adjacent to the shower sheds, Lady Wanda supplies her crew with a sizable A-frame cabin known as the Sofa Room. Television-less, but stuffed with board games and lined with windows, the Sofa Room has become, either out of respect or necessity, the solarium lounge for many of the tired Patients in need of a cushioned respite at day's end.

Into the Sofa Room, Pickers both past and present have placed various "healing" artifacts. The shelves are lined with miniaturized busts of the Venus of Willendorf, Buddha, Shiva, Ganesh; tin chickens and earthenware piggy banks; brass candle-less candlesticks and polished water-less river rocks; a salt-and-pepper shaker depicting a morose Roman-nosed planet Earth reclining in a celestial armchair; Kokopelli charcoal-drawn on a sliver of sandstone; rusty horseshoes and red sequined burlesque garters; coconut shells painted to look like fish; ceramic fish painted to look like gods. It's a silver-haired new-age guru's wet dream and a midwestern cynic's excuse, first, to perfect his eye-roll, but then, because he feels guilty for being intolerant and judgmental (maybe this is where the Jewishness comes in), to nod and smile, and, overcompensating, accept the fact that he has a lot to learn.

I first met Crazy Jeff and Gloria in the Sofa Room one night while searching for Pictionary. Johanna and I had long been fostering an addiction to the game, and it was in our characters to throw, on occasion, one of the drawing pencils across a room in a fit of excitement or frustration. We had convinced Lance to be the all-time drawer so Johanna and I could play one another.

Gloria was sleeping on an orange love seat next to the board game closet, her head teetering between her own shoulder and Crazy Jeff's. Crazy Jeff sat next to her, staring at the exposed wood ceiling as if the beams were tea leaves.

At this point, somewhere into my first week at Weckman Farm, rumor had it that Crazy Jeff was a former cocaine addict who still had the occasional lapse, and Gloria was a paranoid schizophrenic. The rumor went on to speculate, in a nervous-excited whisper, that although Crazy Jeff preferred men, he took Gloria as his lover in order to live off her social security checks.

Many of Weckman Farm's crew members thrive on perpetuating and adding to the fictions of their coworkers. Perhaps the temptation to make legends of themselves for a pair of newbies is too much to resist. Perhaps the realities of farm work, when taken hour by hour, are just too mundane.

Crazy Jeff, we came to discover, was never a coke addict, though he did cop to a few dabblings. Gloria, while eccentric, does not have paranoid schizophrenia. They have become wonderful friends, but they are not lovers. Crazy Jeff and Gloria are both Patients, living with HIV and numerous unnamed afflictions for fifteen and ten years, respectively.

Without breaking his gaze from the ceiling, Crazy Jeff cleared his throat and said, "Only Scrabble's left, ha, ha, ha, ha, ha!"

Soon, while Gloria slept—her black hair stiff and straight, her nose wailing like a pennywhistle—Crazy Jeff and I began talking about how Lady Wanda paid him for his work.

Crazy Jeff (called *Crazy* because of his frequent bouts of often-unprovoked maniacal laughter) told me, "I get a little over three grams of the good stuff an hour. Like an ounce a day. For this stuff, that's like five hundred bucks! A day!"

Approximately 85 to 95 percent of Lady Wanda's seasonal yield will be sent on to medical marijuana hospices and dispensaries, sold at "retail prices" (about five hundred dollars an ounce). The remaining 5 to 15 percent goes to pay workers like Crazy Jeff on a collective basis. The rest of us, of course, are invited to toke from their joints.

"Can you believe that?!" Crazy Jeff cried. "There's nothing more physical than physics!"

Of course, he then descended into a disturbing bout of giggles, which he staunched, as if hiccups, by meditatively rubbing the cysts that plague the undersides of his ears. Each cyst is about the size of a halved wine cork, and Crazy Jeff often keeps them covered with circular Band-Aids. For this reason, some of the less kind of the Pickers refer to him as Frankenstein, an insult Crazy Jeff is prone to dismiss with a wave of his hand and a sharp, singular "Ha!" He's in his late forties and, though balding and unwell, he looks young for his age. I never amassed the courage to ask him about his laughing, the reasons behind it, but Johanna theorized that he took the "laughter is the best medicine" advice far too literally. He aggravated her far more than he did me.

He shifted in the orange love seat as his laughter subsided. Gloria woke up, disheveled. She looked at me, then Crazy Jeff.

"Whaaaaat?" she demanded.

LANCE IS PART of the second group who chooses to be paid in pot, a group Charlie the Mechanic affectionately dubs "The Bud-Fuckers."

"That's all they do. They fuck bud. The sonsabitches love their weed more than I do," Charlie would say, the tone of his voice struggling to be heard through an electronic-sounding rasp. Lance would often counter by accusing Charlie, being a mechanic, of reconstructing his own throat with a series of screws. Charlie would counter back, "You got it, little man. And fuck yourself."

Lance and his fellow marijuana enthusiasts, ranging in age from eighteen to seventy, choose to be paid solely in pot for the sheer enjoyment of smoking some "really exotic stuff. Connoisseur stuff, man. Real delicacies."

So as I said, in not so many words, Lance is a beautiful man, blessed with feminine features, a jawline so sharp it could double as a letter opener. I think most of us on Weckman Farm were drawn to him in one way or another. My own attraction to him can best be characterized as lustily platonic, if I can get away with that. Ogled by crew members male and female, gay and straight, Lance is the fun-loving target of equally fun-loving harassment. He is the blonde-haired, blue-eyed demigod of countless teen idol pinup magazines, his lazy, pot-fueled speech easily mistaken for a confident drawl. Like a photo, his face is glossy and permanent. Like the often-photographed, he's come to depend on the attention it garners him.

Lance claims to have grown up in Southern California, near Pasadena, but these claims are often mumbled and unspecific, and Charlie the Mechanic routinely dismisses them as bullshit.

"The boy's a surfer wannabe," Charlie would say, "but he ain't never lived in Southern California. He's always been here."

Lance would counter this with a stunning silence, during which he swayed all listeners to his side.

It was by means of Charlie the Mechanic's ridicule (which I'd like to believe was good-natured) that Lance earned his third title, one he wore like a badge and bragged about. Lance the Field Manager. Lance the Head Trimmer. And Lance, King of the Bud-Fuckers. This was how he introduced himself to Johanna and me—yet another crew member stoking his legendary status, earned or unearned, I couldn't yet tell.

AT THE DINNER TABLE, Crazy Jeff is holding up a baggie that must contain twenty freshly rolled joints.

"Whoo-hoo! Whoo-hoo-hoo!" he cackles to no one in particular. "Funny cigarettes!"

Charlie the Mechanic is in the middle of telling Johanna, "Boutros Boutros-Ghali is the Antichrist."

Sadly, I didn't hear how this conversation got started. As a matter of fact, most of this dialogue is half-remembered by a half-stoned guy who wrote many of his notes in the Coleman Cimarron tent after dark, without turning on the lantern and risking disturbing his slumbering wife (pardon all the -ing words there).

"Uh-huh," Johanna musters.

"And I am the Sun God!" Charlie follows, to the delight of Lance.

In my notebook, in crooked blue Papermate after-dark handwriting, my note of Charlie's strange claim borders on the illegible. *I am the Sun God* could easily be *I am So Good*, but why would I have made it a point to write *that* down? Plus, Charlie would say things like that all the time, situating himself in the realm of mythology. According to my notebook, he also once said, unprovoked, "I got lightnin' in me!" but I'm not certain how to work that into the story.

Lance high-fives Charlie and I finally chime in, "I don't know what the fuck any of you are talking about."

If I had to guess, I was a little stoned, and Johanna was too.

Hector smashes a mosquito against the side of his face with an audible slap. He laughs at me. "Dude, it's the end of the day. Who does?"

"Well . . ." Gloria says.

"So. So," Crazy Jeff interrupts, trying to get my and Johanna's attention, "I'm sitting in Trax [a Haight-Ashbury bar] and the bartender puts down three drinks in front of me. And I look around . . ."

Here, Crazy Jeff looks around Lady Wanda's carnival dinner tent with eyes and mouth agape. The twenty tables surrounding ours are holding their own courts, filled with their own din, and the soothing sound of plastic silverware clicking against a chorus of teeth. At one table, an unseen male voice, with a slightly Germanic accent, bellows to his giggling audience, "I am a *doctor!*"

". . . and I say to the bartender," Crazy Jeff continues, staring wide-eyed at the center of our rust-painted picnic table, surely envisioning those three glorious drinks, his voice growing louder, "I say, 'I didn't order these.' And the bartender points to three different guys in the bar and I think, This is the curse! This is what my father was telling me about!"

As if on cue, Crazy Jeff falls into laughter and begins rubbing his cysts. Then, he points with one hand to three different tables under the tent, mimicking the bartender's long-ago indication of Crazy Jeff's triple appeal. He's smiling like a boy. We all laugh with him. I feel shell-shocked and look to Johanna to see if she feels the same. She shrugs with her eyes, but she is laughing. I feel the urge to hold her hand with my right and Crazy Jeff's with my left. Instead, I use my hands to slap my legs, hoping that this gesture will allow me to laugh harder than I am. I think it actually works.

Hector shakes his head, a tiny explosion of blood holding to his cheek where he smashed the mosquito. I wonder if Hector is thinking about "the equivalent."

When Crazy Jeff ends his crazy laughter with an exasperated "Hoooooo," the table goes quiet for a moment. In this time, the night temperature seems to drop ten degrees. Johanna kisses my ear in a way that's pleasurable in its wetness, and painful in its loudness.

"Well," Gloria says.

Three

IN THE RESIDENTS' CAMP, rain and digestion. It's pushing midnight, but still, Johanna and I are captivated by our stomachs, engaged in a croaking call-and-response symphony likely spawned by Antonio's corn cakes. We're huddled in the center of our Coleman Cimarron tent, trying to stay dry as the weather knocks at the side walls.

We listen to the camp's shutting-down sounds—the series of "goodnights," the zippered closings of the final few tent doors. I can tell that for me, sleep is still a long way away. I have a head full of pot smoke, and it's beginning to ache. This does not bode well; tomorrow is a Cutting Day.

Earlier, as Lance, Crazy Jeff, and Gloria enjoyed their after-dinner joints with Johanna and me, and Charlie the Mechanic licked the last of the herb sauce from his paper plate, Lady Wanda made her nightly cameo appearance. For such a large woman, she has a way of appearing out of nowhere, as if a fat-fetishist magician's assistant, emerging from a cloud of barely legal smoke. Tonight, she graced us with one of her tighter tank tops—the red one that has become a joke among some of the crew members. This was, of course, before the rain.

She loomed over Charlie, as cumulous as the gathering clouds, her planetary bosom keeping time with the earth. Part of me (the deviant part) wanted to plunge headfirst into her cleavage and reemerge with a giant nipple in my mouth—something to do with a hazy brew of sexuality, warmth, comfort, protection, womb, shame. Hell, most of me wanted to do it. Instead, I quietly kissed Johanna's ear. Before Lady Wanda spoke, she placed her hands on Charlie the Mechanic's shoulders. Charlie leapt, his tongue retreating from his paper plate back to its proper lair as if he were just attacked by a pair of nail-polished biscuits. A hush fell over the collection of rust-painted picnic tables, the mish-mash of stories finding their space breaks.

"Sleep well, my babies," Lady Wanda announced, "for tomorrow is a Cutting Day."

Cutting Days, as Lance had informed us in his infuriating, desirable manner, involve grooming the crops to encourage further growth. Just before breakfast, we were to meet at a converted tractor shed toward the east side of Lady Wanda's house. Here, we Pickers would each be given a set of pruning shears.

"The earlier you get there," Lance told us, "the better the shears. My advice: go for the ones with the blue handles."

We were to follow Lance to a designated segment of the crop. Here, we would find, attached to each plant by a rubber band, a number written on a paper tag. These numbered plants were to be cut about two inches above the base, whereupon we would be put to the task of hewing through each branch and cutting off the large outermost leaves, each about the size of a baseball mitt finger and held to the center branch with a thick stalk. We were expected to complete this supposedly rigorous task with the delicacy required to keep the marijuana buds undamaged.

"Thank you, everybody," Lady Wanda said, and whirled from the dinner tent, bounding like a cue ball for her mansion.

When she was out of earshot, Charlie the Mechanic crumpled his paper plate in disgust.

"This is bullshit," he complained. "I worked another farm where the Pickers just picked. They had Cutters for the cutting and Fanners for the leaves. And she expects us to do this in a day?"

"It always works out fine, Charlie," Lance crooned, his experience at Weckman Farm asserting itself in his voice.

"Fine for her, I'm sure," Charlie said. "But this is stupid. She just doesn't want to pay for a proper crew."

He looked to Hector for a measure of support, but Hector just shrugged.

"I'm up in my tree sunrise to sunset, man. Don't look at me."

"That's why your dick looks like a little piece of bark," Charlie growled.

Hector swatted at the air. "That's *redwood* bark, man."

As if in the rear of a junior high school bus, big dick/little dick jokes thrive on Weckman Farm.

"I'm done with these small farms," Charlie said. "No fuckin' Cutters, no fuckin' Fanners. Pretty soon, we're cooking our own food."

Fanners earn their names because of the toughness of the stalks that connect leaf to branch. On many other farms, Charlie assured us, the Fanners are supplied with electric machines that resemble a square of chain-link fence impregnated with rotating fan blades. His explanation though, was punctuated with a lot more *fuckin's*.

"And she has us doing it with clippers. It's just fuckin' stupid," Charlie whined.

"Easy," Lance said. "It works every year, it's energy efficient, it's . . ."

"It don't do nothin' for my energy," Charlie interrupted.

Lance just shook his head. Crazy Jeff and Gloria had already left for the Residents' Camp or the Sofa Room. Hector stood up.

"Can't listen to any more of this," he said, the blotch of now-dry blood still holding to his cheek.

I looked at Johanna. We followed Hector, walked with him in silence to the Residents' Camp.

The crops, from their privileged position atop a small hill, taunted us with the thickness of their stalks. Surely, there's a dick joke in there somewhere—my ticket to belonging. The fields tonight, encased in shadow, darker than the sky, looked like a lot of work.

"I'm out," Hector said to us, unzipping the flap of his eight-person tent.

As soon as he was inside, the rain began.

JOHANNA'S STOMACH SAYS something in Esperanto. Anyone can understand what it means. Her trip to the portable bathroom takes her into the withering pulse of the Residents' Camp. I leave our tent with her, stepping into my damp shoes. The rain, while cold, feels good. Now unburdened of the desire to stay dry, I am graced with the sight, for the first time this season, of a silent, peopleless Residents' Camp. Everyone tucked inside their tents, the camp holds to the dirt like sixty beached manatees still slick with the ocean. Nothing more than a community of sodden tents looks so much in need of saving.

I try to imagine my parents out here, roving like polar bears in search of their seal dinner, my father, like Johanna, shunning any food that didn't once have a heartbeat (he's stubbornly been on the first stage of Atkins for almost a decade; yes, for almost a decade he's eaten only meat and cheese); my mother disapproving, even with her dwindling team of white blood cells, of a farm of this sort, and its varied (but all unreasonable) lifestyles.

I watch Johanna run to the row of eight portable bathrooms, each the size of a walk-in closet. She chooses, as always, the second one from the left. She thinks that it's consistently the cleanest. I think that she's starting to go crazy. I listen to the rain and the first set of snores arising from the far end of the camp. One of the manatees is beginning to moan. It must be Charlie the Mechanic. Perhaps, in sleep, he's having trouble with tonight's dinner as well.

EXCEPT ON THE worst days, my mom insisted on cooking for my dad, Johanna, and me, even through her treatments. I mention this because my thoughts invariably stray to food, not because I want to milk what I promised would merely be the backdrop for my story. My obsession with food may be the only reason Alex, Emily, and Antonio are getting as much press in this tale as they are. Minor character plus food equals major character.

It would be something simple—matzo meal pancakes with crappy maple syrup, chicken she could throw into the oven and forget about. Anyhow, if this sick mother thing is disturbing you, picture her cooking in a yellow bandana with FUCK printed in red across the forehead. And if you wish to point out that a mother who so vehemently shuns the smoking of pot would never, *ever* wear such a bandana, then kiss yourself on the elbow. You are right. The bandana was actually one worn by the famous Native American artist R. C. Gorman whenever he would come for lunch at the Taos, New Mexico, restaurant I worked at a few years before these events. The bandana served to keep autograph hounds and disingenuous fawners at bay, lest they interrupt his afternoon bender on by-the-glass Sterling Merlot.

Every Thursday, Johanna and I would wake up to a house populated only by my parents' three dogs. My dad, earlier in the morning, would have driven my mom to her chemotherapy sessions, and Johanna and I would wait for their phone call. So began the tradition of Chemo Breakfast. There wasn't a shiver or a vomit, a fever or a migraine that could keep us from our sides of ham and crispy hash browns. In my family, food—breakfast most of all—was our ticket to acceptable selfishness. We could commit most crimes short of murder and, to each other at least, justify them with a simple "I was hungry."

At eleven o'clock or so, we would get a call from my dad, impressive in its concision.

"We'll be at Granny Annie's in ten minutes. Meet us there."

Since the owners and staff of Granny Annie's are engaged in an operation that is entirely legal (unless serving weak coffee is now punishable by law), I am using the restaurant's real name. I can not tell you how liberating this is. I've never been good with secrets, and have been prone to blurting out people's birthday gifts in living rooms and kitchens across America.

Telephonically, my dad would leave us no time to ask how my mom was doing, to ask if she was really up for this. He's one of those people who hangs up the phone without saying good-bye. This drives me crazy, as each time, I end up saying a few last words to an empty connection and am answered only with the mysterious hisses and burbles of unseen wire.

Johanna and I would give the dogs their various medications and

31

treats, each of the three having a distinct ailment and palate that came to define our morning routine. Eyedrops and a pig's ear for Juneau, eardrops and a liver snack for Bear, Vaseline on the nose and a piece of stale bread spread with plain Greek yogurt for Kodiak. As Charlie the Mechanic would have said, these were high-maintenance motherfuckers. The dogs' names are also accurate since their many illegal activities can be explained by the fact that they're dogs.

Granny Annie's was a biscuits 'n' gravy sort of diner that became such a comfort to the family during my mother's treatments that we developed a shorthand for our favorite menu items. Skirt steak and eggs became "Arrr!" This exclamation was to be spoken like a pirate, which was how my dad initiated the abbreviation.

Arrr! Steak 'n' eggs! Yes, good clean fun.

Ham-off-the-bone, my father's usual meat option alongside his jalapeño and cheddar omelet, became HOB. The ham was so delicious that its nickname became a synecdoche for both Chemo Breakfast and Granny Annie's.

When it looked like my mother was having a bad Wednesday, the often-asked question was, "Are we still doing HOB tomorrow?"

My mother would muster an "Of course," and burp a plume of chamomile tea. These would rival, in their disease-fueled intensity, my father's infamous Diet Coke burps. For these reasons, though I embrace most edibles from durian to grasshopper, I tend to shun, on most occasions, anything chamomile and anything Diet Coke.

My parents would usually arrive before us. Johanna and I wanted to see my mother already sitting, instead of weaving, postchemo, through the tables and booths to the confusion of the other patrons, even if she were wearing that FUCK bandana. At the beginning of her treatments, when she started losing her hair, she would be slumped into our usual back booth beneath a disheveled wig, my father sitting open-faced next to her. She looked like a mugged transvestite strung out on raspberry wine cooler. I remember thinking that at the time, and even jotting down the comparison on a Granny Annie's napkin, next to a butter stain. As the treatments progressed and she accepted the side effects, she would, now wigless, eat two bites of her breakfast (blintzes or oatmeal) from beneath a pink cancer hat (sorry to change the image on you) clinging tightly to her head, lending an obviousness to her baldness. We would talk about what we were going through to our favorite waitresses, looking for anyone to whom we could unburden ourselves, confess. Johanna and I were two subghosts within this ghost family, impervious to much of the world, and sometimes to each other. As such, when we ate and drank and made love, even in my old bedroom, under the gazes of Ryno and Alyssa and the King Kong hologram that reflected the sun in the mornings, the air mattress making way too much noise, we did so with an intensity that pushed us further into ghosthood. Spitting at death became a hobby, and a vivid one, and one that, according to Johanna, clearly depleted my *chi*.

So my family treated food as salve, as celebration, as birthright. Well, meat, really. When Johanna and I announced our engagement, it was at Gibson's Steakhouse. When it was my dad's birthday, we ate roasted lamb shanks. My family, for generations, wore heart disease, diabetes, and abandon as badges of honor—the stuff that distinguished us from the neighbors. Eating anything that once had a bone, let alone an entire skeleton, was, for my family, like blowing out the candles on a birthday cake. We took the term *transfat* literally: across fat, beyond fat, on the opposite side of fat. How can that be bad? Depending on the context, it could even mean skinniness. Of course, it could also mean really, really fat. Most of us toed the line, dying in our sixties, or, if we took care of ourselves (because we're a vain bunch), our early seventies, but that's like some George Burns shit in my family. My Uncle Murray was legendary for being a Frank male who made it to seventy-*six*, but he was widely reviled for his miserly tendencies, and given his eating habits, those liver spots on his head could have been made by actual, if wayward, chopped liver.

But my mother's affliction was something else. This had nothing to do with the comfortable territory of saturated fat and clogged arteries. We had to fight this the only way we knew how. Food would turn cancer into ceremony. We would make sure of that. Turn this into *transcancer*.

Just before Johanna and I left for Weckman Farm, my mother took a turn for the better, as evidenced by her renewed ability to finish an entire blintz at Granny Annie's. This let us know: it was time for Johanna and me to step out for a little while, see what would happen—to us and to them. This decision did not come without a lot of speeded-up heartbeat.

When we heard that the meals at Weckman Farm were predominantly vegetarian, I (if not Johanna) was pleased. I wanted to remove myself as much as possible from the self-destructive habits of my family, from so much as a drop of fat, from what is probably my inherited nature. After Chicago, harvesting the marijuana crop was the sort of risk into which it seemed easy to escape. Johanna and I would regain our sanctuary, not in solitude, but in a communion that was decidedly not in my family's style: in healthy eating habits; in hard physical labor on the fringe of legality. This is how we thought, and high-fived each other like teenage ghosts on that nighttime swing set.

THE SNORES SUBSIDE. Johanna runs from the bathroom quickly, annoyed by the rain.

"What are you doing out here?" she asks me.

"It feels good," I say.

"You're going to soak the tent," she says.

She's right. My hair is hanging in strings. The rain whispers against this nylon village like a swarm of cicadas. I wonder who of the crew is getting wet, who's staying dry.

Johanna and I crawl in. Our sleeping bags are clammy, but dry. The Cimarron is new, having first expanded its belly here in the Residents' Camp. Weckman Farm is all it knows. I am jealous.

"This sucks," Johanna says.

We lie down on the outside of our sleeping bags, pull two blankets over us.

"Try to sleep," she says. "It sounds like it's going to be a hard workday for you. Okay?"

"Okay."

Johanna throws her leg over me. I think about lifting it, kissing the back of her knee, but I remain still. My stomach is calming down, and the rain is more persistent. Soon, by her breath, I can tell that Johanna is sleeping. I close my eyes but keep envisioning plates of ham, omelets with too much cheese.

I really want to sleep, to wake up early, to secure a set of those blue-handled shears that Lance was talking about. The weight of Johanna's leg is wonderful, a massage in itself. I listen to the rain lighten, then intensify, and lighten again. Our tent keeps everything out. *The crops must be having a field day*, I think to myself, and smile.

"The crops must be having a field day," I speak aloud into Johanna's hair, wondering if she'll hear it in her dream, dismiss me a phantasmal dumbass. I watch the sky grow light through tent canvas, the rain devolve into a drizzle.

I don't mind working tired. Tomorrow's just a Cutting Day, in the middle of a cutting year.

Four

NONE OF THE other Pickers joins my bitching about inflamed arms. Maybe they're used to it, or maybe I have an allergy that my pediatrician never tested for (I don't think ganja was on Dr. Goldman's "scratch test" checklist, somewhere between *eggs* and *ragweed*), but working with marijuana plants, as is the case with most farm work, I've found, is a rash-inducing affair. It's a pulsing, venomous sort of itch, as intense as the smell, a bite from a lawless mosquito. I itch from knuckle to elbow. Maybe this is my karmic comeuppance for shucking a mainstream legality. As Lady Wanda never tires of assuring us, what we are doing may be popularly shunned, "but it is not illegal." I'm not sure if the crew is morally intact or delusional, but like most folks engaged in controversial activity that potentially helps others, we are, if nothing else, fabulous defendants.

In 1996, the state of California passed what became known as the Compassionate Use Act. Under this proposition, patients deemed "seriously ill" by their doctors can legally obtain and use marijuana to relieve their symptoms. The proposition defines "serious" loosely, citing illnesses that range from AIDS and cancer to anorexia and migraine headaches. My favorite open-ended illness is "chronic pain," which is, if one can locate a benevolent and trusting physician, left to the patient to define. I have this hangnail that just won't go away. I have anxiety about getting another hangnail. Don't get me wrong: Johanna and I wouldn't have engaged in such work if we didn't believe in its benefits, but that doesn't mean that the attendant rhetoric is above reproach.

According to the act, the patient's primary caregivers are those who, "And I quote," Lady Wanda would shout, "'possess or cultivate marijuana for the individual medical purposes of the patient'!"

Here, Charlie the Mechanic would lean in and whisper in my ear, "We're fuckin' doctors."

Nothing in the Compassionate Use Act discusses the way a marijuana branch can resist the blades of even the sharpest scissors, or how the work of a Picker can cause hour-long spasms along the palm's life-line, or, most important, how the plants can initiate "the itch."

Usually, this affliction is temporary, fading an hour or two after I leave the fields, while I prepare myself for another one of Alex, Emily, and Antonio's healthy dinners. I wonder if this Picker side effect plagues other members of the crew. I wonder if I'm just a big baby from Chicago.

I sip from my second cup of coffee, barely retaining consciousness under the food tent. I know I'm tired when I daydream about drooling. Charlie the Mechanic and Johanna sip from theirs, also nodding to keep awake.

The Residents' Camp began rustling very early this morning, the tents shuddering like flags at half-mast, memorializing our tragic lack of sleep. If I had an auditory hallucination, it would have involved a bugle and a dirge. A few took showers before work, only to regain their filth in the fields. I fell asleep at what I guessed to be four in the morning. I woke, rashless, at about five. Johanna, not required to report for duty until ten o'clock (the first official work break of the day), got up with me. The sky retained the bluishness of night, a corpse coming back to life. I felt an unholy communion with the sky at this early hour, we coconspirators in zombiedom.

"This sucks," were Johanna's first words of the day.

I was unsure whether she was referring to the ungodly hour or to the dampness of our pillowcases. While the tent kept most of the rain out, we learned quickly that when one is living outdoors, nothing, not even 100 percent money back guaranteed double-stitched seamless vinyl, is waterproof.

I muttered my first words of response. They were 100 percent money back guaranteed unintelligible.

I raced into my shorts and T-shirt and unzipped the tent door, fastening my belt as I walked. I quietly marveled at my own efficiency, then chastised myself for low expectations.

"Good *morning!*" Johanna called after me.

I turned around, walked just as quickly back to the tent, and, bending to the door, kissed her on the lips. I know exactly what that accentuation of *morning* means. Now, I chastise myself for skewed priorities.

"Thank you," she said.

I resumed my heated pace. I wanted to get to the converted tractor shed early, to secure those coveted branch clippers with the blue rubber handles. Lance sold them so well last night. From the Residents' Camp, I walked sleep-chilled (or lack-of-sleep-chilled), across the stretch of ballerina grass dotted with white thimble-sized wildflowers. Is that too precious? Should *ballerina* and *thimble* show up in the same sentence? I'll have to attach to the wildflowers some drug reference, I think. Let's try this: To the center of each, a pool of dew clung, the community baths for the stoned ants and other things unseen.

I passed the white food tent, under which our first meal of the day had yet to be served. The tangle of picnic tables looked quickly abandoned, testaments to a once-thriving colony now resting in ghostliness and dust and decrepitude. Redwing blackbirds walked their tightropes—the roof-seam of the food tent, the volleyball net's upper deck. I'd never seen anyone playing a game of volleyball on Weckman Farm; perhaps the grass surface was too hard for California bones weaned from easy access to beach sand.

Shuddering over this stretch of grass was an expensive-looking riding lawnmower, green and gold with the curves of a sports car— the manifestation of some small-dicked gardener's midlife crisis. Helming this locomotive was the strange looking fellow who Charlie the Mechanic not surprisingly called the Lawnmower Man. The Lawnmower Man, sixty (or so) years old and fixed on his work, would rarely acknowledge the presence of us Pickers.

Sometimes, he might peer from under the brim of his white fishing hat, his gray beard catching the wind like a magic carpet, and stick out his chin as a way of greeting his fellow humans, facial-hair first, his hands never leaving the steering wheel. As always, he was dressed in a black, Asian-style nightgown that just covered his knees. His bone-white calves poked like popsicle sticks from beneath the embroidered hem, his feet reaching into the shadows between the gas pedal and the brake.

"You know, I wonder if he wears any underwear," Johanna asked one morning at breakfast.

I shook my head and shrugged.

Charlie the Mechanic, taking the question seriously, said, "Don't know, but rumor has it he's gotta real Portobello under there."

It was Lance's turn to shake his head.

"Shiiiiit," he said. "You're terrible."

"A baby's arm," Charlie assured us, and began fist-fucking the air above him.

Crazy Jeff just laughed while Gloria stared at the uneaten food yellowing on her plate.

On the grass in front of the volleyball net, the Lawnmower Man's nightgown stood its ground on his thighs, the garment appearing to be as heavy as a lead radiation vest. I quietly thanked the gods of X-ray and *plumbum* and trudged toward him, the man in my path to the tractor shed. I wish I could tell you I caught a glimpse, could confirm or deny the rumor. But while I'm certainly not to be trusted, my memory of Mendocino County is cracked like the Liberty Bell, and I can't lie about a guy's penis. Johanna thinks I imbue my own with far too much importance anyhow. But that's a story—a series of stories—that should, and will, remain, disturbed and titillated, in my childhood bedroom.

My heated pace invigorated my confidence. Despite the Lawnmower Man's penchant for unrequited salutation, I mustered the courage to wave to him. The lawnmower lurched toward me, daring me into a game of chicken. I was up for it. I took another step forward, the tractor shed calling me from a distance. Never before had I been this close to the lawnmower and its man, this twenty-first-century centaur with the placid face of a Buddhist monk. Or maybe he had the body of a monk and the face of a centaur. Anyhow, choose the version you find most compelling. (I'm privately going with my first instinct, a lesson learned from twenty years' worth of multiple choice tests.)

My palms began to sweat, perhaps in response to my closeness to a rotating blade, perhaps in anticipation of an entire day closed over the handles of indomitable branch clippers.

I looked to my white gym shoes and pictured them in tatters. I looked to my right hand, stunned to see it raise itself without my bidding and dare to wave a second time. Above me, a flock of indistinct black birds came together in a perfect ring, wedding the sky. This is true. I remember those damn birds. Johanna routinely chastises me for paying more attention to things like leaves and crows than to what actual people are saying or doing. I wondered if, to them, those damn birds, I was a certain victim, future carrion. I watched in horror as my hand remained erect, fingers luring this cyborg into some kind of response. Above me, one of the black birds cried out, and the remainder answered. I envisioned myself cut into bite-sized pieces. Chewing gum in the grass, resin-flavored and spicier than cinnamon.

The Lawnmower Man, as usual, angled his chin upward, but at this proximity, I could hear his voice over the engine, maybe saying "Hi" or "Hello," but reaching my ears as more of an abstract "hhaaaaaaaah . . ."

I lowered my hand and exhaled through my nose. This incantation from a famously un-incantatory man was my triumph. The warming day was my trophy, topped with a gold-plated Mulching Lawn Hog. If marijuana sterility is a myth, I hope to sire a few offspring to whom I can pass on this metaphorical trophy. If it's not a myth, I'll excise these last three lines from this book, depressed and emasculated.

I had no doubt that, at the tractor shed, Lance would bless me with the tools of my choice. The Lawnmower Man shoved the steering wheel to the left, heading up the mild slope toward the crops. I couldn't help but wonder what the man's voice was like without the engine drowning it out. Above me, the disappointed birds flew off, searching for their brunch elsewhere.

At the tractor shed, ten other Pickers had the same idea, camping out early to claim the best clippers. This was the barnyard version of trying to get front row tickets to a Bruce Springsteen concert. Lance sat shirtless at the back of the shed on a beam of wood anchored into the rear wall. He had a tan the color of a penny, a comparison further enhanced by the tattoo of Abraham Lincoln's profile on his left shoulder. The sixteenth U.S. president faced inward, as if divining the afflatus for his next important proclamation in Lance's left nipple.

Lance's feet dangled above the ground and he kicked his legs like a seductress from a diving board, a refugee from a stylized advertisement for button-fly jeans. My brain went to Phoebe Cates in the pool scene in *Fast Times at Ridgemont High*. I began wondering if it should worry me that Lance was the catalyst for this but then decided that such worries are irrational. I'll take any route to Phoebe I can get, though I'll admit, if I didn't have the same 1980s history with her that Judge Reinhold's character had, I'd be much more inclined to fantasize about Bollywood darling Aishwarya Rai.

A pair of mating wasps circled Lance's feet, skating figure eights on the air. That may not be true, but it may be. Lance is the type of guy who inspires all living things to couple. I'm sure, though unseen, the amoebas were having a killer sangria orgy. As I stepped into the shed, the floor littered with skinny nails, sawdust, and bird shit, Lance emancipated himself from his perch. He sang his song.

"Clipper time," he intoned.

Again, Lance's self-love here was slightly annoying, and I annoyed myself by buying into it, allowing him ego inflation. I am an enabler. I let this guy feel important because he distributed cutting tools. Was

I that entrenched in the context and values of this place? Was I just way too tired to think straight?

Stamping his feet, Lance yanked a cardboard television box away from the rear wall and began pulling out the premier tools.

"These are the best. Who gets 'em, who gets 'em," he called like a drowsy auctioneer.

"Right here, brother," Charlie the Mechanic piped, reaching forward with his right hand.

Lance passed the clippers to Charlie and Charlie tested his purchase—the weight, the spring action, the palm-feel.

"Hmm," he said, offering his appraisal, "Not bad. These'll do if they hafta."

He patted me on the shoulder as he turned from the shed.

"I'll go see what we're havin' fer breakfast," he said.

"Step up. Who's next? Step up," Lance said, segueing from drowsy auctioneer to tranquilized barker.

Inspired to assertiveness, called to the sideshow, I reached my hand through the crowd, wiggling it like a fish. A set of blue-handled clippers found my palm. I gave them a squeeze. The spring was taut but yielding, the blades sharp, the rubber warm. They were a perfect fit. I stood there in my exhaustion, sensualizing the clippers that would carry me through the day. In my hunger, I made mental comparisons between the clippers and other tailored items: *gloves, shoes, bowling ball . . .*

Working on a farm, you quickly learn to assign names and personalities to your equipment. Most everyone on Weckman Farm did it. So I'm only mildly embarrassed to admit that I named my tool "Clippy," and in my mind rescued "him" from a life of performing black market circumcisions at the Israeli consulate in Tijuana.

Charlie the Mechanic called his "Nigel," after the former tool of a nefarious Parisian marine biologist named Dr. Deep Wataire, who used the cruelest means possible to implant radio tracking devices into the brains of great white sharks.

"He was a bastard," Charlie would say about Dr. Wataire, "but a badass risk-taker."

At this early hour, I was jealous of the history of Charlie's clippers. It was a better story than mine was. As I've already said, and will likely continue to say, Weckman Farm is a place of inflated legend-making. Blue rubber handle dangling from the front pocket of my shorts, I made my way to the food tent. The lawnmower, the Lawnmower Man, and the sound of the lurching engine were nowhere to be found.

Johanna was sitting at our usual table with Charlie the Mechanic. At this hour, Hector perched from his post in the treetops, eating his usual granola bar, using his rifle as a crutch and balancing stick. I wonder if he mimed Chaplin up there, mimicking the dancing dinner rolls routine from *The Gold Rush* with a pair of .300 Win. Magnum bullets. Crazy Jeff and Gloria were taking the Cutting Day off. Lance had yet to distribute the lesser of the clippers. Surely, in the realm of Weckman Farm, and the smoke-filled heads of the crew, these were laced with tetanus and gangrene.

Johanna had Charlie laughing about something. They had both filled their plastic red bowls with pineapple muesli, today's delicacy. Alex, Emily, and Antonio had decided to do nothing more culinary this morning than open a box. Or maybe, as I had so often heard Antonio accuse Emily and Alex, the two of them were "too busy making out in the walk-in!" I filled my bowl, grabbed an iced-down bottle of water, and streamed my coffee into a styrofoam cup from the thermos spigot. It smelled good—like weak earth and waking.

"What's so funny?" I asked, sitting down.

"Oh, shit, brother," Charlie managed. "Yer wife's got some nasty stories."

I turned, confused, to Johanna.

"The obese amputee," she said.

"Unbelievable, brother. And it seems like such a luxury job," Charlie said.

"Yeah," I said, "not so luxurious."

Johanna was referring to an instance early in her massage career. She had a regular client who used to work at a small airport, and who had lost both legs after being run down by a Cessna airplane.

Though he was legless, he still weighed, Johanna estimated, about 370 pounds.

"And he really needed the bodywork," Johanna would say, "but he never showered before his sessions, which I think is pretty disrespectful. When I performed certain strokes with my forearm," and here she would mime the stroke along her hip, "I would come up with an armful of this old gray soap scum."

I could only imagine Charlie the Mechanic at this point of the story, running his hand over his sandy stubble and crying, "Oh!"

"And one day," Johanna would continue, "I was massaging his back—and my therapy room at the time was tiny, about eight-by-four—and, just as I lean into a stroke, he lets rip with this tremendous fart . . ."

At this point, I could only imagine Charlie the Mechanic slack-jawed, a lone muesli oat holding to his lower lip.

"And it's horrible. I'm doing my best to press on, to stifle my gag, to be professional. And then, just when it starts to go away, he turns to me and says, 'Johanna, would you mind stepping away from the table so I can let out a really good one?'"

"No . . . *way!*" Charlie must have bellowed.

"Not really glamorous at all," I confirmed.

"Sick-ass shit, brother," Charlie said. "I'd rather be out pickin' any day."

"Me too, I think," I said.

By the time I finish my second cup of coffee, Lance steps into the food tent, his blonde hair trailing behind him like a bridal train. He's now wearing a shirt. A red linen button-down. A shirt on Lance is as incongruous as a bra on Brian Bosworth. That simile is all for the sake of its tongue-twister qualities. It was between that and an iron maiden wearing lingerie. Somehow, I regret both as insufficient. In a previous book, I made another regrettable comparison, discussing the incongruity of an energetic Italian chef sitting down as "a roadrunner taking a nap." It was only after the book went to press that I found out that roadrunners often enter into a nightly torpor during chilly nights in the desert. Apparently, I am leaving a trail of unreliability behind me like crumbs. Stale ones.

"About twenty minutes," Lance calls to the Pickers under his command. I make an O of my lips and exhale loudly.

"I hear ya, brother," Charlie says, then turns to Johanna. "Better bring yer nose plugs," he says.

"Right," she smiles.

I inhale the bottom of my coffee cup and chew a few grounds. Cutting Day. On an hour of sleep, I need all the fuel I can get. I'll spare you the butane reference . . .

IN THE FIELDS, four deer stand in a rectangle eating at the plant tops. All true.

"Hyah!" Lance calls to them, waving his clippers as if stirring a horse to a gallop. Half true. It wasn't a horse, but a buffalo, and it wasn't a gallop, but a lumber.

The animals raise their heads in unison. You may be picturing deer, horse, and buffalo now. Isn't that sort of fun? The early sun yellows their short fur. Obviously unthreatened, they saunter toward the rear of the fields, disappearing into the trees, their bellies full of pot leaves. Surely, their day will be spent in a blissful, tie-dyed herbivorism. Lance tells us that this is a typical problem.

"If not the deer," he says, wind inflating his red linen shirt, "then the chipmunks or the raccoons, or the bugs."

"Or the DEA!" Charlie the Mechanic chimes in.

"Yeah," Lance says. "We have a lot going against us out here."

Soon, we Pickers find ourselves alone in assigned rows, using our carefully named tools to cut the designated plants. I open Clippy's mouth just wide enough to fit the thumb-thick stalks inside. My embarrassment over the name *Clippy* is now starting to expand. Just so you know. I'm aware. Blinking sleep from my eyes, I grip the blue rubber and, with a morning strength that singes my forearms, pump the handles repeatedly with both hands until the stalk is cut through. This takes quite a few pinches, Clippy's teeth surely filed down to the nubs.

46

The wood is not completely dry, still somewhat green and elastic. This does not make for easy work. By the time I make my way through two of the numbered plants, the calluses on my right hand begin to open up. The rubber handles, which earlier had seemed so warm and yielding, now turn on me, tightening, hardening, like belt leather. The sun crests the trees and inflames my pores into an admirable sweat. Well, admirable to the CEOs of Procter and Gamble. As Johanna had instructed me, I begin to stretch between each cutting, calling upon the lofty and the low for strength; I salute the sky, then the earth, the sky, then the earth, shaking the soreness of tent-living from my shoulders. Here, at paragraph's end, I'm wondering if that Procter and Gamble reference was too obscure. Deodorant. That's what I was going for. Deodorant. A futile weapon against the wares of Weckman Farm. Here, even Secret is PH unbalanced.

Lance tells us that, on average, these are large marijuana plants. Depending on elevation and weather, each plant can produce anywhere from six ounces to a pound and a half of usable marijuana. Given that the buds are featherweights, this accounts for quite a mass.

Each main cutting has about eighteen to twenty-five smaller braches that need to be separated. I hold each of these branches to the sun, watching the buds glisten, hairy, the color of wet brick. The large outer fan leaves stretch open as a talon, rescued from prehistory, and mustering the determination of a paleontologist, I slice the drier of these leaves off with the multitalented clippers. When trimming the buds, we are instructed to leave a couple inches of branch attached. I fall into a clipping rhythm that, were it not painful, would lull me to nightmares.

From this elevation on the crop hill, I can see the neighboring cattle ranch, one white longhorn running from the herd, a mere ping-pong ball on the horizon. Even at this distance, I can see its loose skin slithering over its bones. And beyond the ranch, a small cemetery, headstones like playing cards about to topple; a life and death game of Go Fish. Here, Northern California's privileged rest quietly with pink sea salt in their lungs.

Though the ocean is close (sometimes, listening, I can't tell if that's the Pacific or the wind), it remains hidden in all but sound and smell. The air here stinks of brine and marijuana, a circle of hipster shrimp, a skunk with evolved flippers delivering its stench to the coral.

Charlie works two rows ahead of me, cutting his way through the plants before breaking to mount his tractor. He pulls double duty today, many of the Patients choosing to rest. He expresses his fatigue in audible groans that resemble a dishwasher on the fritz. His breath is a study in overacting.

"Uuugghhh," he exhales, "uuugghhh, uuugghhh . . ."

Already, I'm hungry, developing a taste for red grapes dipped in maple syrup—the fresh and the sweet and the tannic. I imagine Johanna back at the Residents' Camp showering in the now-quiet tent village, preparing for ten o'clock and her first massage of the day. Perhaps she's slowly sipping a cup of coffee with Robbi the Yogi.

When Johanna first came to the United States from Sweden, she came with Robbi. The two of them, wishing to shed the Arctic, flew into Miami and eventually migrated to Key West, where they found work in a community Laundromat. I was working as a waiter and assistant sommelier at a local restaurant and met Johanna at three o'clock in the morning in a Latin jazz bar called Virgilio's. My advice to you is: Do that.

She kept ordering me mudslides, even though I told her I never drank them. Though I never drank them, I drank every one. The sweet and the fresh . . . On this, I am finally reliable. (I think I may have blown my load there. Wouldn't that have been a nice last line for this book? Hell, maybe it will be anyway.)

Robbi doesn't spend her nights in the Residents' Camp anymore. She met a six-foot-eight-inch displaced French Canadian who owns a house in nearby Fort Bragg. They often get their breakfast at this shanty called EggHeads, which, according to Robbi, boasts a museum-worthy exhibit of *Wizard of Oz* memorabilia. Robbi is all about, *Oh my God!* As in: "Oh my God, Johanna, you have to come there with me! The crab omelet with champagne hollandaise! Oh . . . my . . .

48

God!" If you heard her speak, you'd know the exclamation points are not excessive. In fact, in limiting myself to one per sentence, I am the Earl of Understatement.

Robbi now sleeps beneath that most endangered of species on Weckman Farm: four walls and a ceiling. Now, she dreams next to a giant man whose legs get cut off at the knee by the foot of his bed.

"As a yoga instructor," Johanna assures me, "I'm sure she has interesting ways to navigate the guy."

Even if Robbi is a little piece of gristle, the way Johanna says this, almost whispering, inflames what Dana Carvey's Church Lady would have called my "bulbous tipping region."

As I approach the stem of Plant Number 34, I'm not sure I have a way to navigate this—the trimming, the cutting, the season, the tent, the swing set, the Patients, the West, the Midwest . . .

BY EIGHT-THIRTY in the evening, ham-off-the-bone doesn't seem so evil anymore. I have filled a crate with the marijuana buds, piled atop one another like a bacchanal of illicit pinecones. I use *bacchanal* because it's one of my mom's favorite words. She teaches eighth grade English (they call it *Language Arts*, as if it entails sculpting busts of Johnny Tremain with prepositional plaster and a palette of past perfects), and rarely has a chance to use it.

Though all of us must be starving, Lady Wanda predicts only our thirst. She huffs along the rows, dropping thermoses of coffee, six-foot styrofoam cup towers, bottles of cold water. She is a medicine ball blown uphill, calling, between heavy breaths, "You're doing, *whheew*, great, all of you. *Whheew* . . . You're *angels*."

Even my halo is hungry.

"Fallin' by the minute!" Charlie the Mechanic calls, his voice detached, crashing, unseen behind his row of plants.

"Remember," she calls, ignoring Charlie, "the meaning, *whheew*, of our work. Make the world, *whheew*, a better place."

A litter of shitty activist songs mewls in my head, suckling on the hypothalamus.

Lady Wanda litters us with refreshments, aphorisms, and breath-lessness, and disappears.

If I am an angel, my wings are killing me. I drop Clippy to the soil. After a couple hours of work, my tool has shed its winning personality, and I want to send the blue-handled fucker back to Tijuana to face his fate. Somehow, this repetitive (the optimists would say *meditative*) work forces me to think way too much about Chicago. This trip to Weckman suddenly seems hasty and forced and incorrect, having stemmed from a decision made with a ghost brain and see-through heart. If this is only a stage in our lives, suddenly it seems like the backstage at a rock concert, unglamorous and littered with sawdust and set paint. But if Mick was right and we can't always get what we want, hopefully what I need is a sore hand and steady buzz. Is it ridiculous to ask for more? I mean, if we are the world, I want Pluto back. If we are the children, I want my mom.

The sun continues its cruelty. I walk to the row's end, watching Lady Wanda's mansion come into view over the greening slope. I swallow two small cups of coffee and a bottle of water. All traces of last night's rain have steamed away, the sun unhindered in its desire to heat. I trudge back to my row, the numbered plant tags vibrating in the hot wind. I try to use my limited ability to add and subtract, to lessen the length of my assigned row by some miracle of arithmetic. Nothing Pythagorean can save me from this. Retrieving Clippy from the dirt, I resume the cutting, my palm blossoming with an enviable bruise.

"String boxes coming in!" Lance shouts an hour later, positioning the massive cardboard boxes at the end of each row.

When she brought our coffee, Lady Wanda mentioned something about this step, but I wasn't really listening.

"What's the story with these again?" I ask Lance.

"Mold, man," is all he answers.

I think of blue cheese, smack my lips.

I carry my crate of marijuana buds to my assigned string box. They bobble as I walk, push their perfume to my nose—a blend of deer breath, black Tellicherry peppercorn, and parsley. The smell is the epitome of *fertile*. Cow shit birthing a rose; iceberg lettuce in heat. The smell alone seems to harbor the potency to heal cancer, or if nothing else, to provide the comfort of the absent-minded — hand-picked manna from hospital heaven.

The string boxes look as if they once housed refrigerators and the technicians who built them. Peering over the cardboard lip, I see a tangle of white yarn crisscrossing the width of the box at various heights, a mess of spider-webbed diagonals, adhered to the sides with scotch tape. M. C. Escher's monkey bars.

Lance spent his very early morning constructing these makeshift drying chambers, the soft-drug version of arts and crafts, a world of underground lanyards and neon popsicle sticks.

Lance reiterates, "No mold on Weckman Farm."

Charlie the Mechanic clears his throat. He wants to say something but remains quiet.

Next to each string box, Lance places a cylinder of small paper clips. These are to be the primitive tools of the curing process, a method by which the marijuana buds are slowly dried. We're told that a good dry can last anywhere from two to eight weeks, depending on the percentage of moisture in the bud. This step ensures that the crop has a long shelf life, a pleasing taste, its intended healing properties. It also ensures that I must make some mental leap between reefer and office supplies.

Moisture in marijuana, an effect of elemental exposure, can, if improperly handled, spawn an outbreak of mold, ruining the crop in both flavor and medicinal value. It was pathetic to imagine, after all this work, these browning rabbits' feet leaking their luck.

"Nobody ever felt better by suckin' on a spore," as Lady Wanda says.

If the cut buds are stacked atop one another for long periods, the unfortunate bottommost layer may fall victim to such an outbreak. It is for this reason that Lance, his hands ginger, his linen shirt now unbuttoned, steps to a string box to demonstrate. He throws his head back like a burgeoning Robert Plant, as if waiting for an offstage floor fan to lend him the look of the fashionably windblown.

The crew walks to the ends of their rows, meeting in the center pathway that Charlie sometimes calls Tractor Alley.

"When I'm drivin'," he would say, "ya best look both ways before crossin' Tractor Alley."

I found this keen advice to heed.

Lance holds an oval of marijuana between his thumb and forefinger, baiting our curiosity. He looks like an elementary school teacher, the alphabet strung behind him, about to launch into a unit about caterpillars and butterflies.

"Okay," he announces, his voice thickening, "fasten, *carefully*— that's the key word—a paperclip to the branch piece at the end of each bud. You may have to loosen each clip a little so it doesn't pinch too tightly, just tight enough to hold it. Then, starting at the bottom of the box, attach it to the lowest string, so it hangs upside down."

"Ornaments on a Christmas tree," Charlie interjects.

"Yes. Thank you, Charlie," Lance says.

"My favorite ornaments!" another Picker shouts.

"Okay, okay. Mine too," Lance confesses, his youth and authority dueling for advantage. "Um. Now . . . String each bud about a half inch apart. Work your way up, lining 'em along each string . . ."

"Like a clothesline!" Charlie yells, pumping his fist in the air. He's obviously delighted with himself.

"Smoke them clothes!" the other Picker cheers, snapping his suspenders, Charlie's sidekick in disruption. I'm quietly delighted at these class clowns. Lance undermined is a more tolerable Lance.

"Right," Lance affirms. "Uh, line 'em along each string until you fill the box. Simple as that. Then, Charlie, you're gonna tractor 'em in for us?"

"You know it, brother."

"Okay. Let's go at it for another hour or so, then break."

Like sewing, this work requires deftness and a love of the eyelet. I allow my forearms to relax, the tendons to uncramp, as I string each bud from its umbilical branch to the interior of the giant box.

When I was waiting tables in Key West, I found my meditation in opening side-work: folding napkins, polishing wine glasses. I find this again. I imagine myself a beekeeper for the crippled and the wingless, hand-populating the hive. When I come to a large bud, I think of Johanna's obese amputee in insect form and want to tell Charlie the Mechanic of my little meditation. But I don't have the energy to explain.

After an hour, I have strung the box half full.

Lance calls, "All right, let's break," from the downslope of Tractor Alley. He has tied his linen shirt over his head. He looks like a Foghat groupie, lacking only the hood of a Trans Am on which to park his ass.

Walking downhill to the food tent, where we are promised crostini spread with Vegemite and local butter, I wonder how many people have completed such work without the benefits of red meat. Right now, it's not a protein *substitute* that I'm craving. I crack my knuckles and stare back up the hill. The marijuana plants stare back, focused. Somewhere, on the other side of the ridge, the longhorns and the headstones welcome the afternoon.

I WONDER HOW many people will feel better because of what's in these strange webbed refrigerator boxes, and the tired people who filled them. We shuffle like the damned into the food tent. There's something very factory-worker-on-a-lunch-break-as-initiated-by-the-wailing-steamwhistle about all of this. We should be covered in soot in lieu of soil. Maybe it's my dinosaur fetish reasserting itself, but I remember thinking of the opening credits to *The Flintstones*.

I've read that Fred's catchphrase, "Yabba-Dabba-Doo" (in the days when catchphrases were still cool, and an essential component in getting a show on television), was a bastardization of the Brylcreem ad slogan, "A Little Dab'll Do Ya," which suggested that a minimal blob of water–mineral oil–beeswax mayonnaise would be enough to hold any Rudolph Valentino hairdo in place while adding enviable gloss. Perhaps Fred started to use the phrase when, going on his own lunch break at Mr. Slate's quarry, he realized that even as he slid feet-first down the tail of his prehistoric beast of burden, his hair didn't so much as flutter in the breeze. Was this catchphrase created by a series of lazy animators who simply did not want to redraw, frame-by-frame, Fred's windblown hair?

Another theory behind Yabba-Dabba-Doo is a bit more felonious and, thus, more appropriate to Weckman Farm. Yabba (often spelled *Yaba*) is a fusion of caffeine and methamphetamine, popularly known in Thailand as *crazy medicine*. It comes in the form of orange or green tablets and is often coated with artificial candy flavors such as grape or (my raving techno grandmother's favorite) butterscotch. Dabba, in Marathi (a language of western India), refers to a cylindrical box, typically constructed of aluminum or tin, often used to enclose complete lunches or spices. Doo is obviously slang for shit, but further research reveals that in this case, it may be shorthand for doo-wop, the beloved voice-heavy version of rhythm and blues. So what was Fred saying as he slid down that brontosaur's tail (it may not have been a brontosaur—it's tough to tell with a cartoon)? Something akin to "I've Got the Methamphetamine Spice-box Blues!"? Is this where Bob Dylan derived some of his inspiration, adopting his cryptic persona because he didn't want to demystify himself by citing Fred Flintstone, his contemporary, as a source? Is it any wonder that William Hanna and Joseph Barbera, producers of *The Flintstones*, created a decidedly trippy "anti"-drug PSA in 1970?

Conspiracy theories aside: we eat, rescued by simple food, Alex the chef our *dabbawalla* today. We go from damned to blessed in no time flat. The butter is fantastic—a reward in itself. The bread, too. Something in me, for the first time in my life, thinks about quoting the Bible. Maybe I'm feeling guilty for slandering, even if only in my head at the time, Hanna and Barbera, those lovely souls . . .

"This is all organic stuff," Alex announces before we eat, hoping we all pause to bow our heads to the holy trinity of spelt, wheat, and oat.

"I toasted the sesame seeds myself," Emily says, her shoulders back, her breasts pushing against Alex's arm, as if an actual—and not figurative—electric charge holds them together.

They exemplify the hippie chic, the ubiquitous look of Northern

California. Alex, a lanky six-foot-two, has a calm face, a survivalist in repose. His raggedy beard belies his trendy horn-rimmed glasses, his DKNY shirt, his expensive Dansko chef's shoes made to look inexpensive. In appearance alone, Alex is the epitome of *nice*. Turn-the-other-cheek *nice*. Grit-your-teeth-and-nod *nice*. But he smells like food—like garlic, and cumin, and mustard seed. Usually, that's enough for me.

I know I asked you to dismiss Alex and Emily as—how did I put it?—"pseudohippie wallpaper." But they are a specific kind of wallpaper—plaid and shiny and stinking of old glue. A little like my childhood bedroom wallpaper, the kind that Johanna called "the dark side of retro." The kind that, as we kissed in its ambiance, gave me both sleeplessness and peace.

During our first week on the farm, before the rigors of the job sent us to bed early and reinvented first impressions, I gravitated toward Alex, Emily, and Antonio; they reminded me also of my past life in the restaurant industry. Alex and I began to talk over a couple bottles of the North Coast Brewery's Red Seal Ale. (This was one of the few times alcohol penetrated Weckman Farm. "You hear about the violent drunks," Lady Wanda would say, "but you never hear of someone beating their wife because they smoked a joint.")

Before meeting Emily in culinary school, Alex spent over a year in India, a third of that time in a hospital.

"For some reason one day, I just fell into a stupor and didn't come out of it," he said. "Cold sweats, vomiting, diarrhea, sleeplessness—the whole nine yards. I thought it was something I ate—a safe assumption, you know? Eventually, I had to go to a doctor—this old Bengali man with something like a British accent, but more regal, you know? He took one look at me and said—I'll never forget it—'Mistah Ahndrews, you have . . . mahlaayyriaah.' It was so drawn out and dramatic. You know what I mean?"

Perhaps, Alex's face is more worn than calm—that of a man who has fully accepted the wildness of the world. Still, he was full of "you knows?" and he spoke them in a way that let his listeners know that none of us would ever really know what it was like to be Alex, even though we were also being forced to nod affirmatively. I would never really understand what it was like to be him, waking delirious in a Calcutta hospital, the sounds and light there, what the floors were made out of, what was hanging on the walls, the temperature at night, whether or not his doctor wore glasses, the hushed, accented voices diagnosing as he daydreamed. And he would never know that I held, behind my noddings of *yes, yes,* the experience of weeping with Johanna in that stupid Buffalo Grove bedroom, thinking we would never be able to leave, that mortality had become the mistress that would forever change the way we loved each other, defined our marriage; Johanna and I regressing together in that small room amid drawers concealing old junior high yearbooks in which girls, trapped in time, had scrawled "Have a great summer" in obese bubble letters, and boys had fused, in chicken-scratch, the newfound linguistics of "summer" and "fuckin' great." When we're asked "You know what I mean?" and we answer "Yes," aren't we always lying?

Though about the same age as Alex, Emily appears much younger. She often cooks in a flowing purple skirt, anchored to her waist with a braided rope of lavender and gold thread, tiny tarnished bells attached at each end. She's incredibly well-spoken, perhaps having garnered her impressions of the world from great literature instead of the malaria ward of a Calcutta hospital. She is barely blonder than Alex, her cat's-eye glasses more tapered. I see her as a hippie Charlotte Brontë, having exchanged her Yorkshire pudding for pot. They are beautiful nerds who have found their niche.

Antonio stands silent behind them as they offer their organic blessing over their organic bread. He wears a white apron over a white T-shirt, and baggy black pants studded with stylized chicken drumsticks. His shirt's sweat stains are impressive, oversized amoebas pushing from beneath the apron, the color of Darjeeling tea. His ample gut must have housed enough lard-laced tortillas in his fifty-something years to render such an epicurean swell. Though he must have twenty-five years on Alex and Emily, he stands pouting behind them, the scolded child in their kitchen.

"The Vegemite," Alex continues, "is Antonio's contribution."

"I'm Australian," Antonio says, eliciting the small laughter of a tired, nearly humorless picking crew.

The trio of chefs turn from the food tent to the kitchen. I watch Antonio put a hand on Alex's back, trespassing on Emily's property.

"You know, if I was you, boss," he says, "I would just let them eat without saying anything."

A serene look stretches over his face as he says this, his hands folded over his bulging gut like two ethereal, Euclidian trapezoids.

Five

ACTUALLY, IT'S WE who eat without saying anything. At least when we start. Charlie the Mechanic, sitting across from me, dips his head to his plate, genuflecting to the creamy saltiness of the crostini. His sidekick in disruption sits next to him, wearing a turquoise windbreaker over his red suspenders. He looks like a ballooned sixth grader, looks like he should be standing at a school bus stop, strapped into a backpack, picking on a smaller kid. This is the first time he's infiltrated our table, the lunchroom clique of Johanna and me, Lance, Charlie, Hector, Crazy Jeff, and Gloria penetrated for the first time. Though the entire crowd isn't here today, the sidekick's presence is unnerving. I can't help but recall Ricky Meyer, can't help but recall that recollection is tough on bullies, shoving (as if Ricky itself), the memory of Paul Yu finally standing up to him in the gym locker room, throwing the headlocked Ricky, and his reputation, over his hip.

In the fields of Weckman—as Charlie can attest to—you can make and lose friends quickly. It's like adult recess. The sidekick's name is Bob. He must be in his late forties or early fifties and has the beet-red face of a man who has spent a lot of time on sailboats, in a tank top bearing a sexist fishing slogan, drinking his beer from the can. I imagine him to be the type of guy who loves showing off his armpit hair, as if it defines him as a concentrated bullion cube of masculinity.

Rumor has it that he used to be a cop in a rough LA suburb, but his alcoholism got him fired; that he bounced around maintenance jobs for apartment complexes and condo associations before landing on Weckman Farm. He's probably come here to dry out. Exchange one vice for another. Bob is the first to speak.

"This is pretty good," he manages through a mouthful of crumbs.

"You got it, brother," Charlie affirms.

"I tell ya, I'm not looking forward to going back out there," Bob mumbles. "Bending over that string box has my back in a shambles."

"Go see his wife for ten minutes," Charlie says. "She's magic."

"Oh," Bob says to me. "It's *your* wife who does the massage?"

"Yeah," I say, nodding, knowing before he says anything else that I'm going to have to defend Johanna and her occupation. My heartbeat quickens. I think of kissing her ears on that air mattress in Chicago, smelling her neck in our tent.

"Shit, man, more power to ya," Bob says. "If I was married, I wouldn't want my wife doing that, y'know?"

I hate it when people react this way to Johanna's job, spewing obviousness and ignorance and obvious ignorance—as if every barman were a pimp and every massage therapist a whore. I feel the blood rush to my face, my stomach sink. My body wants to punch Bob, but I try to calm it down. I am becoming Paul Yu without the biceps.

"Why is that?" I ask.

"Well, you know," Bob chortles, looking to Charlie for support.

Charlie looks up at me from his crostini prayer and shrugs his eyes. He offers Bob no support and I want to hug him for it. Bob is the type of guy who depends on the worst kind of male support, while remaining relatively harmless. Charlie, in his silence, has debullied him. Bob is naked. Bob is weaponless.

"Well . . . I don't know," he says. "If you're fine, I'm fine."

"I'm fine," I say.

Bob goes back to eating in silence, and I can't help but feel a little bad for him. He clearly doesn't want to make enemies. He doesn't know about my quickening heart, Johanna's ears, Johanna's neck, my father's coughing, my mom's Telly Savalas imitation . . . I try to make conversation.

"So you used to be a cop?" I ask Bob.

"I did, yeah," he says. "A while ago." He jiggles his gut up and down with both hands, indicating that he used to be in much better shape.

"So does it ever seem strange to be working in this industry?"

"Well," Bob considers, "what we're doing is pretty much legal. Technically. What the dispensaries do with any of the leftovers is, well, up in the air."

"But I hear of the police busting up farms anyway. Lady Wanda says that the farms don't get any governmental support in these instances."

"Well," Bob says, "there's so much that's official and so much that's unofficial that the line is pretty much blurry. Plus, every time a new suit takes office, new little technicalities are added to the law. No cop has the time to keep up. And nobody cares. It's not like we're doing church work and we know it. Everybody knows what we're getting into."

At this, my heart drops a little in my chest. I start to wonder just what exactly Johanna and I think we're doing.

"Parasites," Charlie says, wiping Vegemite from his lips.

"Huh?" I ask.

"Parasites," Charlie repeats. "The suits, brother."

"Oh." I turn back to Bob. "So why did you leave the force?"

If Bob is seeking entry to our mealtime cabal, I at least want to get to know him, to confirm or dispel the rumors; to hear the legend-making from its source. I don't remember if it happened right then, but the wind would often whip his windbreaker like a sail. The sound was often the loudest thing within earshot, and in that small moment, Weckman Farm could have been an ocean, and we all could have been riding something easily capsize-able. On its deck, like a low-rent Beethoven, Bob would be standing, armpit hair unfurled, waggling his prick in defiance at everything more powerful than he. Of course, he would be the first to drown.

"A couple reasons," Bob begins, affecting a well-practiced tone, his voice crawling like a groundhog into the deep recesses of his throat, where it finds no shadow and limitless, if false, authority. "First, I was on this team assignment to bust up a heroin ring. And the more I investigated, the closer it led me to the government. First the mayor, then the senators and congressmen, all the way. One by one, my partners dropped off the case. Too much heat from upstairs. And finally, the chief calls me into his office and orders me to lay off the case. 'You gotta let it go, Bob.' And I tell him, 'After all this work? No way.' And he says, 'Fuck you, Bob.' And I say, 'No. Fuck *youuu!*'"

Confirming my Bob-at-the-bus-stop impression, he swears in a way that evokes the same response such language coming from the mouth of a seven-year-old would produce: it's one part funny, three parts disturbing, and six parts the way of the fucking world. I am compelled to mention also that my experience has made me distasteful of anyone referring to their bosses or superiors as "upstairs." As someone who grew up in a raised ranch, in which bedroom and kitchen and living room were upstairs, and the downstairs was cold and dark and scary at night, *upstairs* to me holds the comfort of home, while *downstairs* is the out-of-reach and the washer/dryer, the dog food, the ghost story . . .

Here, Lance enters the food tent from the fields where he has been correcting "Picker errors," as he diplomatically calls them. His red shirt continues to moonlight as a bandanna. He sits next to me, breathing heavily, dropping his full weight to the picnic bench. As he joins the table, the air around us seems to warm, grow younger.

"Gentlemen . . ." he coos.

"Hey, Lance," I say.

Charlie points to him without looking from his plate.

Bob ignores him, never breaking his story, which, to Bob, is the zenith of importance, laced, I fear he may believe, with *advice*.

". . . I'm not laying off this case. So I was fired. Can you believe it? For wanting to do my job."

"That's bullshit," Charlie says.

For a moment, Bob is silent, and I think I may have been wrong about the moral. I likely sighed, relieved. But then:

"Never forget that, young man. It's better to do what you believe in and suffer the consequences than to suck ass."

The "suck ass" part almost redeems Bob's moral from the groan-worthy, but not quite.

"What's the other reason?" I ask.

Lance wipes his nose. One of the newer Pickers, who joined the crew after Johanna and me, brings Lance a paper plate of crostini. She's a redhead—probably eighteen or nineteen—pretty, freckled, and bowlegged, a wallflower on a crooked stem. She looks as if she spent most of her childhood on horseback with Band-aids over both knees. She is Missoula, Montana, in cutoff jeans. She doesn't sit with us or say anything, but it's clear she has a crush on Lance.

"Thank you, Ruby," he says.

Ruby, I think. *That's just about perfect.*

Ruby flits away like a swatted moth, rejoins another table at the opposite end of the tent.

"The other reason's a little more complicated," Bob says, his gaze following Ruby back to her table. "I uh, one day, uh, had a couple drinks before duty and, uh, was called into this assault where this guy ended up at the bottom of a pool . . ."

The groundhog in his throat has crawled forward and, in the rodent-shaped darkness there, is fucking scared. I am wondering which synonym for *groundhog* would suit Bob best—I'm guessing, in ascending order: woodchuck, whistlepig, land-beaver.

Charlie begins nodding at Bob's story, as if he'd been there, or had lived through a similar situation. A dead guy and a pool. To guys like this, older hat than Venus Wear.

". . . and I was the first to arrive on the scene." Bob's eyes start to glass over—tiredness or memory or misery. "Aaand, the guy was pretty young. Twenties or so, and definitely needed CPR. So I started in, you know?"

Bob put one hand on top of the other to illustrate.

"Do you know CPR?" he asks.

"Johanna's certified," I say. "And I learned on that dummy in high school health class."

"Resusci-Annie!" Lance says. "I learned on her too."

"Yeah," Bob says. "Anyways, so you know how I have to pump the chest, then give the mouth-to-mouth and so on."

"Yeah," Lance and I say in unison.

Charlie chews his food. It sounds disgusting.

"So, I give three quick pumps and, well, I just hear, crunch . . . crunch . . . crunch."

Bob pauses, takes a sip of his coffee, swallows.

"So what happened?" I ask.

"Well, I must have crushed his ribcage or something," Bob says and begins to laugh a little.

"Jeez. What happened to the guy?" Lance asks.

Bob just sits there. He's not quite nodding, but bouncing up and down, as if on the balls of his feet, but he's sitting.

I look at Charlie. Charlie nods. Old hat.

"Did he die?" I ask Bob.

"Yeah," Bob says, exhausted, as if the outcome were at once obvious and still a surprise to him.

He emits a sound between a choke and a laugh. He's sipping his coffee faster now, like it's the only way he can swallow, as if the faster he sips, the sooner he'll forget this story. I wonder how faulty his memory is.

"Shit," Lance says, the word for him now holding at one syllable.

We finish our light lunch in silence, all of us bouncing.

At the garbage cans, tossing our paper plates and cups, I ask Lance if I can take a break from the fields to help Charlie load the string boxes into the curing shed on the far side of Lady Wanda's house.

"But the tractor only has one seat," Lance says.

"I can ride on the flatbed. With the boxes."

"Why would you wanna do that?"

"Well, you know. Curiosity. I'd like to check out all facets of the operation," I shrug. Of course, I could not tell him I was planning to write about all of this.

"Well, sure. I guess. We actually got more done this morning than

I'd anticipated. Sure. Sure. I guess it would make my job easier," he says and pats me on the chest. This small affection feels good, brotherly in a way that, brotherless, I can only guess at. If I'm picking weed for a living, I suppose I can get away with ending that sentence on a preposition.

Ruby walks to the garbage can, looking only at Lance. She throws in a paper plate and a water bottle.

"Hi," she says, and scrambles away.

Bob joins us at the trashcan, apparently the crew's version of the office water cooler.

"Who's ready to pick some *weeeeed!*" he cackles, slapping me on the back, moving-on and bliss residing, simply, in loudness of voice and extension of vowel. I wonder if this technique will work for Johanna and me. If we can escape into rhetoric, allow *cancer* to become *can't-cer*, moving-on to have an actual destination. Things to be as easy as words.

"THIS IS THE BAT CAVE," Charlie calls to me over his shoulder as we pull from Tractor Alley to the curing shed. Like most things named after comic book lairs, the curing shed is light and shadow, insect and sawdust, and not nearly as cool as I expected. What Charlie calls the Bat Cave, Lance calls The Enclosure, which is a little more serial killer than comic book. Both names chill my blood, the former to the level of an ice cube dropped into muscadel, the latter to Kelvin.

Charlie cuts the engine and dismounts. I shuffle among the eleven string boxes that we were able to fit on the flatbed. Though awkward to handle, the boxes are reasonably light. Lance charged Charlie and me with loading the flatbed ourselves. Once it was full, I squeezed myself in among the string boxes, and Charlie began his reckless descent along Tractor Alley, ignoring potholes and rocks with equal measure. We bounced along as if on a rickety wooden roller coaster from the 1950s, one in need of a few nails.

As we passed Bob in his turquoise windbreaker, he called, "Red Flag! Red Flag!" and I waved, nearly slipping from my feet and knocking our meticulous string boxes to the soil.

As we passed Lance, he clasped his hands behind his neck, flared his elbows outward, and proceeded to hump the air like a reject Chippendale. Charlie laughed aloud. I remember that: this high-pitched nasal laugh that miraculously rose above the grinding of the tractor's engine. I remember also thinking of a dentist's drill. Despite his position of authority, it was good to see Lance act like a stupid kid. Leaving the crew, we passed a legless scarecrow made of sackcloth, its face composed of wooden buttons and black magic marker, its stuffed arms above its head, signaling victory over all flying things. I wonder if Lady Wanda built it. I wonder which of us on Weckman were the crows.

The rough ride inflamed my back and shoulders, nearly causing me to cough up the crostini. Charlie held the gas pedal to the floor and I spread my feet as wide as I could, praying that I didn't topple from the flatbed. Finally, we shot from Tractor Alley into the mown grass semicircle that serves as the Bat Cave's parking lot. Before he cut the engine, Charlie let loose with a wonderful belch. I don't remember if I smoked anything or not before this wild ride. If I did, it's likely I invented Charlie's belch, but it's something he would have done, saved it for the moment he twisted the key in the ignition, the two bursts of simultaneous energy lending him, if only in his mind, an added gravity, an internal, if not spiritual, power, a kinship with all things mechanical. That's just the type of guy he is.

I elbow my way through the cardboard mob. Its aroma is intoxicating—I feel I am becoming anesthetized through my nose, through the crop oils on my hands. I'm starting to regain my perspective of the world as a still, unvibrating place. I'm starting to question the reality of this perspective. Charlie is at the shed door, unlocking the padlock, before I can hew through the load. His shirtback is ringed with sweat, his hair recalling Raggedy Ann's. With a lighthandedness, he pushes the heavy red door inward. I wasn't close enough to notice his fingernails, but I'll bet they were sensationally filthy.

The Bat Cave is dark, more buggy than batty, though a few bats do hang, upside-down and asleep, from the high ceiling. Likely stoned and thus imbuing Charlie with the role of invincible bodyguard, I fear the bats far less than I normally would have. The shed looks as if it once served as a barn, and still holds a musky, animal smell. Goat or sheep or goat-sheep. By the colonies of insects swarming like stars in the little sunlight that creeps through the roof cracks, the ancient plum stains on the concrete floor, and the implacable stench of old shit and metal, I guess that this building was, in the days before Lady Wanda's rule, used as a dungeon or slaughterhouse. Behind every support beam, I expect to see cobwebbed thumbscrews and stretching racks, iron maidens and scold's bridles. I expect to see Franz Kafka, alive and well in the corner, scribbling into a spiral notebook. That stuff I must have smoked must have been some good shit.

As Charlie and I step inside, spiders scramble to the edges of the room, the bats hang motionless—dead chandeliers that can not, will not, be turned on. In fact, the Bat Cave doesn't harbor a single light, outlet, wire, or window. It's ready for Edison's resurrection. Only here can his inventions once again be new. The room is cool, armored against the sunlight by surprisingly effective clapboard.

Charlie and I will have to work by the light that seeps in the open door and through the cracks in the walls and ceiling. I blink to adjust my eyes. To the left, a series of circular blades rest behind what appear to be plastic cages, certainly a new device of torture, yet to be named. I blink again. They are merely battery-operated box fans.

On the far wall, suspended from thumbtacks, are wire hangers tied with string. From the string, individual marijuana buds dangle, a mobile for Jerry Garcia's baby. Somewhere, in the celestial mono-chordal space where all mothers are allowed clairvoyance, my own is wondering, after a particularly rigorous session of radiation, what her nice suburban Jewish boy is doing in a room like this. Shouldn't he be behind a cherrywood desk spread with embossed papers in a building that is decidedly not-farmhouse, decidedly wired for electricity? Shouldn't he be making love to his wife in a room that bears a private toilet, a shower stall that is kind to bare feet? How the fuck did he end up here?

"The old method, I guess," Charlie explains, dismissing the hangers with a stamp of his foot.

We begin to unload the truck. It takes both of us to handle a single box, the buds thumping the cardboard interior. Trapped roaches. Ha.

"Jes line 'em up along the wall for now," Charlie says. Again, I'm not sure if it was because I smoked something, or because the acoustics of the Bat Cave resembled the acoustics of a bat cave, but Charlie's voice began to sound a bit more abbreviated, his intonation more colloquial. He seemed to have shunned the letter *T*.

It takes us about a half hour to unload the bed. By the time we finish with the eleventh box, a muscle spasm begins in my trapezius, a mouse kicking beneath the skin. This is a comparison not hastily made. I read that the word *muscle* derives from the Latin, *musculus*, which means "little mouse." It seems the Romans thought that the biceps wriggled like mice beneath the skin. In one way, this comparison thrills me; in another, it totally devalues the hero worship I, as a child, thrust upon Lou Ferrigno. At any rate (even the going one), I never imagined that carrying boxes so light could be so taxing.

After lining the boxes against the wall, the square-jawed victims of an imminent firing squad, we turn the twenty box fans to medium. The breeze stirs the constellations of insects, Andromeda blowing apart, Cassiopeia revising her curves.

"The venna-lation's important," Charlie tells me, surely regurgitating something that Lance had told him.

If there is a science to the curing process, Lady Wanda favors the shoestring variety. Here, rolodexes still trump the Internet. Apparently, it works for her. While many experienced growers employ swamp coolers, air conditioners, humidifiers, and dehumidifiers to keep the drying buds at a constant humidity level (about 50 to 60 percent), Lady Wanda seems to achieve the same result with discount fans and a drafty old barn.

For the first two to three days of the curing process, we are to leave the string box tops uncovered, the fans going at medium speed. This ventilation will remove an amount of the initial moisture. As the buds begin to dry out, by day four, Charlie tells me, we drop the fan speed to low and drape newspaper over the box tops.

"We start with the comics section and move on to the hard news," he says.

I'm not sure if that's exactly how he worded it. I'm infamous, to Johanna especially, for screwing up jokes.

Anyhow, when I don't laugh, Charlie says, "Just kidding."

In the fields, Lance instructed us to remove only the drier of the outer leaves, leaving the others to shield the bud. During the curing process, the remaining leaves will become brittle and can be removed.

From these leaves, as well as from all parts of the plant removed during the grooming stage, various degrees of marijuana hash will be made. After the harvest, Lady Wanda will keep a few members of the crew on staff (Lance, I think, will surely be one of them) to extract the resin from the imperfect clippings. The leaves and early discards will contain about 15 percent of the plants' resin production.

"They use the Bat Cave as the hash factory after the pickin's done," Charlie tells me, slowly incorporating, as if on doctor's orders, the Ts back into his repertoire.

Lance and his small cadre will empty the discard crates onto a fine-mesh screen lined with pantyhose. I'm no great fetishist of this sort, but I begin to free associate: pantyhose, stiletto heels, leather straps, cat o' nine tails. I try to imagine the Bat Cave kinky.

"The little resin glands'll slip through," Charlie says, "but the screen'll keep the junk out."

After straining, the granular product will be pressed by hand into small, gummy balls. A number of these balls will then be pressed together and flattened into blocks with a rolling pin. With the medical marijuana, these potent bars of hash will be sent to the dispensaries for either eating or smoking. A real kick-ass Snickers.

"The hash'll really take the bad pain away," Charlie assures me. "And the smell in this room'll be amazing, brother," Charlie assures me, "like a nice piece of fruit."

I wonder, but don't ask, which type of fruit.

Inhaling, I smell more bat shit than anything like a cantaloupe. I stand in a skinny pool of sun in front of one of the fans and quickly breathe out.

"What now?" I ask Charlie.

"Now we bring in another load, but there ain't no rush," he says.

He doesn't have to raise his eyebrows twice for me to know what he's talking about.

He reaches to his white tube sock, pulled up to his knee. From the netherworld around his ankle, he retrieves a sweaty, anorexic joint.

"When in Rome," he says.

I shake my head. "Speak Italian?" I felt really proud of myself for that one, given my hazy condition.

Charlie laughs. "Ya wanna do the honors, brother?"

"Wow, Charlie, how are we gonna be the rest of the workday after this?"

He disregards the question and says something like, "This stuff's the Trainwreck. It's a bad name. The stuff's really mellow. Lance swears by it."

"Well," I mock-hesitate, "maybe just a taste."

Charlie reaches into his back pocket and pulls out a matchbook. He tosses it to me, and even in the depths of the Bat Cave, I catch it in one hand. The matchbook bears a logo of an intoxicated orange cat, asterisks for eyes, stuffed into an empty moonshine jug. Below it, in red letters, reads the phrase "Happiness Is a Tight Pussy." Perfect.

I put one end of the joint in my mouth and strike the match. I imagine the field crew, busy with their shears and paperclips, their cardboard boxes and water bottles. I feel Charlie and I are joining a not-so-secret club. Happiness is this club.

The smoke tickles my lungs as if with a cattail, fills my mouth with the taste of a fungal spruce. Immediately, it goes to my head, my brain buoyant in a tepid pool of cerebral spinal fluid. Happiness is a buoyant brain.

"Whheeww," I say to Charlie. "That's it for me."

"You got it, brother," Charlie says, taking the joint from my fingers.

He wipes his forehead and inhales a massive drag.

"Oooh," he says on the exhale. "You know, in Vietnam, every time I killed a man, I smoked a joint."

This is unexpected. His eyes turn down, as if he's divining his fortune from his untied shoelaces. Or, more terribly, his past. He shakes his head. I don't think he meant for that to slip out. I don't think he wanted to break our spell just yet. He's wondering how to catch himself.

"Oh, brother . . ." he says.

I don't know what to say. I don't feel terribly incapacitated by the one drag of this exotic marijuana, but under even its mild spell, conversation of this sort seems daunting. Does this mean I'm gonna have to talk about my mom? Tell him things I've told only to Johanna? Does this mean I'm going to have to engage Charlie as something more than antihero caricature? I want to be the hard-hearted asshole who responds "Fuck that" to these questions, but suddenly, I'm feeling characteristically (and, Johanna would say, often detrimentally) soft. My train feels a little behind schedule but, luckily, remains unwrecked.

"So they say you used to work on some oil rig in Alaska," I muster. (*Fuck that, fuck that . . .*)

"No, no, brother. That was my older brother. He died up there."

This is getting worse and worse. Or, as the wife of an Illinois mayor once said, actually referring to my mom's affliction, "worser and worser . . ." (whispering, shaking head, eyes down), "worser and worser." That's right: four times. I want to be unspecific about the mayor's town, because they are the type of people who would sue my ass over this.

The sun seeping through the ceiling cracks becomes unnaturally bright—a wormhole in the Bat Cave. I want to crawl through it. I miss the sun. The string boxes seem ready to attack.

"I came out here from Oklahoma, brother. Met Lady Wanda at the Burnin' Man Festival in Nevada."

Charlie takes another drag. A lasso of smoke curls from his mouth, roping an errant horsefly. When I'm silent, he feels the need to clarify.

71

"A big art and music festival out in the Black Rock Desert. Supposed to be about self-reliance, but really, it's just lots of fuckin', lots of drugs."

"Yeah, I know about it. I heard you worked on ice cream trucks," I say.

"Yeah. In San Francisco. This was back in my drinkin' days, brother. You're ridin' with me, so you should know: I can't never drive a car legally for the rest of my life."

"You're kidding," I say.

"Nope. Not to say that I don't. When I was workin' the ice cream trucks, the owner let me sleep in the garage. I never had to drive to work. But I ain't had a drink in six years."

He holds the joint to the minimal light. It's shrunk to the size of a maggot. Emasculated. Impotent. Like us.

"This helps," he says.

I want to ask him about his ex-wife, the only consistent character in the varied rumors of Charlie's life, but after the Vietnam War, a dead brother, and alcoholism in rapid succession, I decide to keep quiet. Enough is enough. Fuck that. At any rate, my mind begins to wander, curls into the dim orange light of the Bat Cave and falls asleep. I have no idea what time it is, or how long we've been in The Enclosure. I have no idea if I rendered that dialogue accurately or not.

Charlie the Mechanic falls forward and catches himself. I realize he is walking out the door, returning to his tractor, a man like a string box: disheveled, makeshift, easily broken. My legs move on instinct. I decide not to smoke this Trainwreck again for a while. It seems to stir depressing topics; pot of the perturbator variety. I do what I haven't had to do since the dark days of Chicago. I muster the strength to face the rest of the day.

ON CUTTING DAY, we dine like midday Hobbits. Second Lunch is served at two o'clock in the afternoon.

Charlie and I board the tractor in a dream-state. When he sees that I fail in my first attempt to mount the flatbed, catching my shorts

72

pocket on the exposed metal edge, he leaps from his seat and offers me a hand. It feels good to be touched, like we're finally friends. I stifle the want to hug him.

"Cain't tell ya how many times I fell offa this thing m'self, brother. Don't feel bad."

At least he's got his *T*s back.

"Okay," I say.

Charlie pats me on the back. I can feel the warmth of his hands through my T-shirt.

"Thanks, Big C," I say, having no idea where the Big C came from.

"What the hell time do ya think it is?" he asks.

I treat it like a calculus question, mulling it over. I hold my breath. Old formulas dance across my brain, hiding somewhere behind the hypothalamus. I remember ditching high school math class, only to show up outside the doorway, at such an angle that the class could see me but Mrs. Huberty couldn't, and flop facedown onto the floor and hump the orange carpet, mistakenly believing that this would finally allow Jaime Gilkowski, both cheerleader *and* poetry editor of the student literary journal, to see me as cool. That's not her real name, but it's close. A fusion, really, of two girls I had crushes on. A fusion, really, that in high school I used as "material," alone in my bedroom, years before Johanna and I returned there.

Suddenly, I am aware of how dry my mouth is, how badly I want a sip of water. How I can't possibly begin to fathom an answer to Charlie's question. I exhale. I think to impress him by repeating the question back to him in Spanish. Dazzle him with a little *¿Qué hora es?* but I don't know how to vocalize that upside-down question mark, so:

"Whew," I say. "Got me."

I smack my lips, envisioning my skull's interior to be like that of the curing shed: riddled with dust and bats, with twenty fans to blow the moisture away.

Charlie groans, and in his chest, I swear I can hear a frog die, deflate under the points of a gigging spear.

73

"Welp," he croaks at last, "we should prob'ly get up inta the fields. Pick up another load."

He twists the key in the ignition. The tractor coughs, phlegmatic, belching emphysema from its exhaust, forcing comparisons with Charlie that, in the interest of restraint, will go unnamed here. Another rickety ride . . .

The daylight has changed, the sun sharper at its edges. We interrupt three squirrels, hunched over a common nut. They abandon their meal, dart from the tractor's wheels. This might have been a benign hallucination. I think I remember one of them wearing sunglasses. In profile, I can see Charlie fixed on Tractor Alley, squinting, his jaw tight, his hands gripping the wheel at a textbook ten and two. This time, he does his best to avoid the potholes and rocks. He shifts gears and takes the tractor uphill. I brace myself, trying to protect my head with one hand while gripping the side of the flatbed with the other. Sitting down, I plead with gravity to be merciful. I feel its force holding me down, the spider web of natural law. The temptation to defiantly shout *Eat me!* to the sky is fierce but, owing to the mellow properties of the Trainwreck, not fierce enough. Anyhow, Charlie would have probably thought, confused, that I was talking to him. And I wouldn't have had the energy to explain.

The sun occupies a mediocre place in the sky—not too high, not too low. While the California clock baffles me, I feel that the Trainwreck has offered me a brief glimpse into Central time. It's a Tuesday. My dad must be driving home from work by now, cursing the rush-hour traffic, turning up the volume on *The Score* sports radio show. He has to get home to take care of the dogs—they need to be fed and walked; he has to make sure my mom is still alive. That's something new. Are we always dealing with fresh cusps until we die? Can't we take comfort in the old hat anymore, ever?

Charlie brings me back to the Pacific with three sharp coughs. I wonder if it's my mother coughing through him, trying to tell me something.

"Hell," Charlie growls, the marijuana asserting itself in his lungs.

I wonder if Charlie has ever seen Chicago. I picture him as a young man, hiding his youth behind mirrored Ray-Bans and a voice that had yet to be destroyed. The young Charlie is holding a gun, walking along Michigan Avenue; as he passes, every stoplight turns into a tree, every building its own jungle. By his eyes, I can tell he's in a place whose name he can't pronounce. He rubs his hands together like Lady Macbeth. It's nighttime and Charlie has just shot, for the first time, a faceless Vietnamese man. He stands surprised at the amount of shots it took to kill him, surprised at how much it hurt his hands. He still has a mother and father somewhere. His older brother is still alive, as yet unbeaten by Alaska. He has yet to fall in love with the wife who will leave him, and is only in the developmental stage of his alcoholism.

Maybe this is the day that sent him, some thirty-five years later, to Weckman Farm; to regift the smoke that allowed him to sleep at night in a tent village very different from this one. When faced with such horrors, what can the body crave but ephemera? What else can we do but harvest it?

"Fuck is everybody?" Charlie calls.

"What?" I shout, straining to be heard over the engine.

"Where the fuck is everybody?" he repeats, stopping the tractor, cutting the engine.

The picking fields are bare. Not even Lance stumbles through, correcting Picker errors. Again, I'm struck with the notion of disappearing colonies. I wouldn't be surprised if I never saw any of Lady Wanda's crew ever again, Charlie and I forced to wander the earth together after some silent Armageddon. My heart goes cold. Where is Johanna? Enchanted, and not so blissfully now, by the Trainwreck, I begin to panic. My palms go wet; it's hard to breathe.

"What's going on here, man?" I ask Charlie. "This is fuckin' crazy."

Suddenly, I feel like his son.

"Aah brother, Second Lunch prob'ly," he says. "Cain't believe it's two o'clock already, though."

My stomach anchors me. The sweat returns to its burrow under my skin. My heart decelerates faster than a one-seat tractor.

"Yes!" I say. "A nice meal can diffuse the H-bomb." I have no idea where that came from.

"What, ya talkin' about heroin?" Charlie asks.

"No, you know. The Hydrogen bomb."

"Ha. Right," Charlie says. "We best get over there."

We take comfort in our familiar table. Johanna, Lance, and Bob are a few bites into their salads—mesclun lettuce and ripe tomato garnished with crostini left over from First Lunch.

"We were wondering what happened to you guys," Johanna says.

I want to kiss her hard, then soft, then hide my face in her neck and never resurface. Making conversation is something I've lost the blueprints for.

"I said you made a break for it," Bob supplies.

"Yep," Charlie says.

I pull a bizarre piece of lettuce from Johanna's plate. It looks like romaine spattered with blood.

"What is this?" I ask. These three words are an effort, but I feel I should remind everyone that I may still be human.

"Speckled trout's tongue," Lance answers.

Given my state, I'm certain I misheard him.

"Heirloom lettuce," Johanna says.

"Yeah," Bob says. "You missed Alex's opening commentary. Sparkling trout tongue with collarbone olive oil."

"*Calolea* olive oil," Lance says. "It's local. Gourmet stuff, man. A real delicacy."

I bow my forehead to my hand, rub my temples.

"What have you and Charlie been getting into?" Johanna asks.

She rubs my back and giggles.

"Poaching the product!" Bob says.

"Just a small try," I say. "Just me and Charlie. In the curing shed."

"Niiiiiice," Lance says, lending the word his skills at elongation. "What did you think?"

"I felt it," I say, "I feel it."

Johanna continues to rub my back. Bob pulls at the breast of his windbreaker, fanning air over what I guess to be an ample crop of chest hair.

Lance says, "Yeeeesss."

Turning to Johanna, Charlie says, "Brother's a lightweight."

"I know," she says, kissing me on the neck.

The touch of her lips sparks some kind of emotional shift. I am inflated with an implacable joy. I want to hug everyone at the table. Tactfully speaking, I want to reach in and take it out. Yes, *that* "it." It's the age of Aquarius.

"Friends and lovers!" I announce, gesturing with the back of my hand.

"Which one am I?" Bob asks, cracking himself up.

"Baaaaaahhh!" I lamb.

I heap the lettuce on my plate, speckled and sparkling. I swallow it with crostini and coffee and lots of water. I am a machine aiming to sober up.

By Second Lunch's end, I feel a little like myself again, but more fragile. My doors can be kicked in with a ballet slipper. Having escaped the Trainwreck with a little whiplash, but with my life, I celebrate this second chance at sobriety by letting the flies remain on my plate. It's a particularly buggy day. I wonder how Hector is doing up in the trees, if he's formulating his dinnertime anti-insect monologue.

"Watchya lookin' at, brother," Charlie asks Lance, who is transfixed with something to his right.

He gestures with his head to Ruby, sitting by herself at her picnic table, in a black Canned Heat T-shirt and jean shorts. She sits with that straight-backed cowgirl posture even as she leans forward, thumbing through a stapled packet of photocopied papers.

"Hell," Charlie says, "Ruby the Newbie. I see she got herself the Communist Manifesto."

Johanna and I laugh the loudest.

We all know this packet of papers very well. Within our first day at Weckman Farm, as she does with all of her new workers, Lady

Wanda distributed this literature to Johanna and me with Jehovah's Witness zeal.

"At your leisure . . ." she instructed, winking, her eye shadow a disturbing gecko green. "This is the mission of Weckman Farm."

"Thanks," we said.

I remember her lack of "You're welcome." In its place, she shook her heavy right arm, her hand in the air, surely summoning to Weckman Farm the beautiful Lethe, the river-goddess of Hades and spirit of oblivion. Lady Wanda's doughnut of a costume bracelet—white plastic with faux emeralds—slipped from her wrist to her forearm.

"I think you'll enjoy it here," she said, turning for her mansion, her housefrock bearing white irises that surely smelled of sweat and Secret.

It was not the Communist Manifesto at all but an outlandish eight-page handbook of sorts, which Lady Wanda cobbled together from God-knows-what sources and titled THE MEANING OF WORK. Flipping through it, while newbies ourselves, Johanna and I looked to each other, with wrinkled foreheads, for help.

"Who exactly are we working for?" Johanna asked.

"Ask your friend Robbi."

Those first few days, we often thought of returning to Chicago, then pictured the jaundiced light of my childhood bedroom, the three dogs barking at 5:00 a.m., my mother in a new mail-order skullcap, and rejected the thought immediately.

As we flipped the pages, our reservations about Weckman Farm and its Martian mother hen spread into smiles.

"This is sort of . . . delightful," I said to Johanna.

"Sort of . . ." she said.

Our clique watched Ruby run a pale hand through her red hair.

"I can only imagine what she must be thinking," I say to Lance. "Or what Lady Wanda was thinking when she put that thing together."

"Actually," Lance dismisses, "she's very well read."

I'm not sure whether he's referring to Ruby or Lady Wanda, but I don't push it with Lance. There is a defensiveness in his voice, albeit a calm one.

THE MEANING OF WORK begins in daunting fashion.

> WECKMAN FARM IS A SEVEN-DAY A WEEK JOB.
> WE HAVE PEOPLE WHO ARE COUNTING ON US
> AND IDLENESS IS NOT AN OPTION. WE ARE
> THE INNOCENT KEYS UNLOCKING
> HARMONIOUS ATTITUDES.
> ALWAYS REMEMBER!
> MAKE THE WORLD
> A BETTER
> PLACE.

"I couldn't get past the first page," Bob brags.

Lady Wanda goes on:

> WE MUST TREAT EACH DAY OF THE WEEK AS SACRED.
> IN IRISH FOLKLORE, EACH DAY CORRESPONDS
> TO LIVING THINGS, TO TREES AND BIRDS.

When first perusing THE MEANING OF WORK, Johanna and I had just set up our tent in the Residents' Camp. As we read, I affected the voice of a British narrator, offering interpretation.

"The homes and those who inhabit them . . ."

Johanna, nervous, fingered the walls of our tent.

"What home?" she asked.

Our first night at Weckman Farm, our tent not yet . . . *ours*, I continued to read aloud from THE MEANING OF WORK, as Johanna, my fellow fish-out-of-water, tried to fall asleep on my chest.

> SUNDAY WITH BIRCH AND BARN OWL
> MONDAY WITH WILLOW AND SANDPIPER
> TUESDAY WITH HOLLY AND TERN
> WEDNESDAY WITH HAZEL (OR ASH) AND CATBIRD
> THURSDAY WITH OAK AND DOVE

It was about here that I decided, "This is sort of . . . delightful."

"Sort of . . ." Johanna said, her voice drifting.

"I like the 'or Ash' qualification."
This was, and is, true.

FRIDAY WITH APPLE AND QUAIL

SATURDAY WITH ALDER AND FINCH

Read, Lady Wanda's musings had the effect of counting sheep, the prayerbook repetition lulling Johanna and me not only toward sleep, but to consolation, in our tent, in the then-new sounds of the Residents' Camp—the breathing and quiet guitars—in our decision to come all the way out here. I ran my hand over her hair.

"Read me one more page," she said.

IN EVERYTHING IS CODE!

WE MUST FOLLOW THE INSTRUCTIONS OF THE HEBREW MYSTICS.

At this point, I could only imagine what Charlie the Mechanic must have thought when he first read Lady Wanda's packet. How many *brothers* he uttered.

WE MUST TAKE THE FIRST LETTER OF EACH BIRD.

B, S, T, C, D, Q, F

THESE LETTERS TRANSLATE INTO THE ANCIENT LATIN PHRASE,

BENIGNISSIME SOLO TIBI CORDIS DEVOTIONEM QUOTIDIANAM FACIO

(MOST GRACIOUS ONE TO THREE ALONE I MAKE

A DAILY DEVOTION OF MY HEART):

THIS IS THE MEANING OF WORK!

"Johanna?"

"Mmm?" she muttered, on the verge.

"I was gonna say, this may require some further decoding," I smiled. "I mean, what the fuck is Three?"

Later, via Google of course, I found that *Three* was Lady Wanda's typo for *Thee*. That would've helped.

She lifted her head from my chest, sleepy and incredulous.

"Is she talking about God?" she asked.

"I'm not sure. I don't think so." God and his relationship to a pot farm?

Johanna's head fell to her pillow. Our tent walls hummed in the wind.

The next day, Johanna performed her first farmland massage; I made my first daily devotion of my heart to a cluster of Durban Poison, learning how to shape the buds with scissors, collecting the trimmings in the crate.

We all watch now, with morbid curiosity, Ruby flipping through Lady Wanda's mission statement, taking her initiation alone beneath the food tent, unaware even of Lance's gaze.

Six

BEFORE DINNER, with Johanna still locked away in Lady Wanda's dungeon, performing her day's last massage, Hector invites me to sit in on his checkup. Should we crew members so desire, we can schedule appointments and solicit general medical advice of the stethoscope, tongue depressor, turn-and-cough variety. For a month during the harvest, a local doctor passes his regular patients to his associate and sets up shop on Weckman Farm. Apparently, the doctor's parents were friends of Lady Wanda's parents, and he provides simple care and generic advice to us wayward souls free of charge. I have to wonder what Wanda's and his parents talked about over Saturday night dinners and Sunday barbeques, how they reacted to the directions their offspring were taking, and if they ever imagined such a collaboration. Anyhow, should any serious ailment arise, Weckman's doctor—who I imagine smokes his share—will put us in touch with local specialists who are not inclined to report our very particular smell to the authorities.

Lady Wanda's house doctor is a young blonde man named Klein. During his month-long tenure at Weckman Farm, he also fills in as a Picker.

"I like this work," he says. "Agricultural surgery." This, also, I wrote down in my notebook. Surely, Klein surrounded this nugget with other sentences, but I failed to recall them, or render them in blue Bic ink.

Klein (or the German Shepherd, as the crew refers to him) pulls a hot pink stethoscope from the side pocket of his blue duck-hunter's coat. He unzips the jacket, the flannel lining and sheepskin collar meeting at the Shepherd's thick neck. The Shepherd is slender everywhere but his neck, as if he had, early in his medical career, volunteered for some experimental injections with swelling side-effects. I imagine a superhero named Neckman, the logo of a bloated noose emblazoned in foil on his chest.

Twisting to the right and left, cracking his back, the Shepherd turns to me.

"It's your mother who had the cancer, yes?"

I'm not sure I like that this is my identifying characteristic on Weckman Farm. I purposefully bite my lip, so the Shepherd sees my reluctance.

"Yes," I say.

"But is it done?"

I'm not quite prepared for this. I wish I had practiced earlier in front of the outhouse mirror, or with Charlie in the Bat Cave.

"She's still undergoing treatment," I say. "But the oncologist says that it's shrunk considerably, that there's now a 75 percent chance she'll kick it."

I pause for him to say something encouraging about percentages, about the word *shrunk*.

"Take off your shirt," he says.

For a second, I don't realize he's talking to Hector. A breeze smooths the confusion, a breeze that smells like sugarcane.

"In my experience," he says, "I've found that oncologists are among the most honest of specialists."

"That's good," I say, wondering what the implications of that are, what that says about brain surgeons.

The German Shepherd pauses.

"It happened to my mother," he says.

"Mine too," Hector groans, having a little trouble pulling his arms from his sleeves.

In an instant, Weckman Farm becomes Support Group. We should

84

be sitting in some low-rent hotel conference room, eating butter cookies from doily-lined platters. Now is as good a time as any to admit: I have no idea if the breeze really smelled like sugarcane. Thank you, Support Group.

"Did she kick it?" I ask.

"For a while, yes," the Shepherd says.

Hector says nothing, pulls his shirt over his head. His hair, as always, is the Rock of Gibraltar, unmoving, the most dependable thing on Weckman.

As is his habit, the German Shepherd curls his lips. He looks like a flossless man who just finished eating a stubborn ear of corn, pressing his teeth together to show the world the pressure his mouth must bear. Though young, still in his thirties, the Shepherd treats the Weckman Farm crew as if he himself had fathered us and we weren't easy to raise. I wonder if, as a child, Lady Wanda treated him like an annoying little brother.

"Aaallll right," he intones, waving his right hand in the air, with his left hand cracking the stethoscope like a whip.

Hector, sitting on the Shepherd's examining table (a large collapsible IKEA end table), shifts, a beast about to be tamed. He flares his hands outward and I can see the small red rope burns lining his palms.

At sundown, Hector dismounted his tree. Despite his crow's nest position at Weckman Farm, Hector is afraid of heights and dreads the sunrise climb and dusky descent with the sweaty fear typically reserved for nightmares. These climbs and descents are made by rope ladder.

"The fucking thing is so damn *shaky*," Hector complains.

The Night Sniper, to whom I've never spoken and rarely seen, replaces Hector, scaling the ladder, silent and swift. The Night Sniper is also ex-military, a man named Waldo (prompting Hector to check his watch at every sunset and endlessly question, "Where's Waldo?"). Since I never really developed a relationship with him, I admit that Waldo is his real name. Anyhow, the "Where's Waldo" joke, however lame, depends on it.

"Fucker was late again," Hector says turning from me to the Shepherd. "Where's Waldo, you know what I mean?"

"I do," the Shepherd answers balefully.

Rumor has it that Waldo, a sometimes-Patient, suffers from epilepsy. Just what you look for in a sniper—equal opportunity gone awry. I'm going to leave it at that, lest I offend even myself.

"But he stops every attack," Hector says of Waldo's fits, "by sniffing this little bag of Ginseng Oolong tea. He swears by the shit. And get this: he calls the bag 'Blue People.' This dude is weird, man."

The Shepherd grits his teeth, shifts the stethoscope from Hector's right shoulder blade to his left.

"Breathe," he instructs.

Hector complies with a healthy inhale.

"Beautiful," the Shepherd responds. "Very good. Crystal clear. You sound like a trout stream."

That is no exaggeration. This is how the man spoke.

"All right!" Hector laughs.

He sits on his hands to prevent himself from swatting at the mosquitoes who are now alighting on his upper arms and chest. His vein-green military tattoos do nothing to repel them, becoming, as is typical, pathetic on an aging, fattening body.

"As for your friend," Klein says to Hector, "there is no connection between the sniffing of tea and the stifling of a seizure. It is psychosomatic."

"He's not my friend," Hector says.

"And 'Blue People,'" the Shepherd continues, "is the actual name of a good-quality Oolong tea."

"Whatever, man, he is *weird*," Hector says.

The Shepherd seems to bring out the child in all of us. Hector is the bully, Waldo the sheepish kid with a secret affliction, the Shepherd the principal who warns us of the mutilating potential of a hurled snowball at recess.

Hector's right hand jumps from beneath him, scratches at a fresh bite on his sturdy left breast. His nest of hair doesn't even shudder.

Shirtless, Hector assumes a posture indicating that the Shepherd has tamed him, this lonely bear with spina bifida, his salmon-catching days long over, preferring now the easy prey of low-bush blueberries.

Earlier, when the German Shepherd summoned Hector to his appointment, he and I were sitting on the grass in the Residents' Camp. We had both gotten off work and I was waiting for Johanna, a perfect G-string of sweat running along the median of my shorts.

"Another day," Hector said.

"Had to shoot anybody?" I asked.

"If I did, you'd probably never see me again," he said. "I thought about shooting Waldo. Fucker was late again! Only five minutes today, but still."

Behind us, Lance carried Ruby piggyback into the crops. She dug her heels into his thighs, trying to make him fall. Too young to take the hint, Lance fought to remain standing.

"Never thought I'd be doing this with my life," Hector went on.

"So how'd you come to it?" I asked. "I know you said something about the Army . . ."

"There's this phrase in Spanish," he said, "about chickens in a henhouse. *Ahora si me la dejaste como un palo de gallinero. Bien cagada!* You know that little stick that runs under the cages? That all the chickens shit on?"

"No," I said.

"Well anyway, they shit on this stick. And the saying goes something like, 'We all live like a stick under the chickens.' But sometimes the shit is good, you know?"

"Sort of like the Spanish version of 'Shit happens'?" I suggest.

"Not so much," Hector says. "But the chickens . . ."

"Hector!" the German Shepherd calls, emerging from his fancy insectile mountain-man tent.

In the Shepherd's mouth, Hector's name sounds like *Hek-door!* His voice is thick-necked too.

Still, even now, Hector's henhouse phrase, which I've pieced together as best as possible from memory, notebook, and Google, remains a bit of a mystery to me.

The Shepherd moves the stethoscope to Hector's chest, hiding the mosquito bite beneath the cold microphone. As instructed, Hector breathes.

"Ahhh," the Shepherd sighs. "Like the sea. Like that scene in *From Here to Eternity*, two lovers indulging in the waves."

That's the Shepherd.

"Yeah. I feel good," Hector says. "I just want to check, you know. You're free."

"Not so much," the Shepherd says. "You're good to stay off the marijuana. Save it for the Patients."

The Shepherd, though (I know from first-hand observation), like any good preacher, does not practice what he, uh, you know . . .

Hector shrugs and puts his shirt on, a black T-shirt with white flowers. The sky darkens, a red line on the horizon like an oven-burn. Lance and Ruby emerge from the rows; this time, she carries him. My stomach bucks. The German Shepherd squints at me, pulls a pair of glasses from his jacket pocket, and puts them on. They are the roundest glasses I've ever seen, and heavy, planetary. With the power of two Jupiters, he stares me down.

"And for you, there's no time now," he says.

He pauses, allowing me to consider this statement, its many possible meanings. Then, as a doctor, he knows his role is often to assuage.

"We all have to eat," he says.

Not quite assuaged, I infer in this a meditation on predators and prey, and how the good doctor has assigned each on Weckman Farm their probable role.

When eating, the German Shepherd takes his meals with his regular group of Pickers, an all-male bunch to whom I never speak. The longer I'm on Weckman Farm, the more I talk to a very few people, the less I talk to most.

The Shepherd, with the stethoscope still in his ears like a bib worn too high, holds the small silver dollar microphone to the sky over the crops.

"Man, I can't wait to . . ." Hector begins.

"Sshht!" the Shepherd says, holding his open palm to Hector.

He arcs the stethoscope microphone from east to west. In this sweep, the sky sheds the last of the daytime colors. I'm not sure if there's more arrogance or poetry in the Shepherd here, or if I should make such distinctions.

Hector quietly thumps his chest with his middle finger. He bends to my ear. On his breath, I smell yeast, a sourdough starter, red cherries turning to bad wine.

"I got a heart like an ocean," he says, surely repeating something the Shepherd told him.

The German Shepherd takes the stethoscope from his ears, replaces it into a corridor of his duck-hunter's coat. He stares at us with a doctor's pity, a hunter who loves ducks but must kill them because they eat his lawn. He knows his priorities are skewed, but nevertheless, they are his. From another of his coat's passageways, he pulls a white packet of diner sugar, opens it, and empties it into his scowling mouth.

"If you listen," he says, swallowing sweetly, his lips dropping like curtains to his teeth, "you can hear the deer sleep."

THAT NIGHT, after a dinner of spaghetti with icicle radish, lemon, and Calolea olive oil, we follow another of Lady Wanda's handbook chestnuts.

RESTING THE BODY IS GOOD
FOR THE SOUL.

Johanna and I recline on the floor of the Sofa Room.

Outside, unzipping his eight-person tent, we can hear Hector shout, "*Pinche* mosquitoes!"

Gloria stretches out on the orange loveseat, teetering between sleep and awake. Crazy Jeff sits cross-legged on a blue pillow, his back supported against the base of the loveseat, his head finding the bony crook of Gloria's hip. He holds the palm-sized Venus of Willendorf sculpture in his fist.

"I think I feel my fertility coming back," he says finally, laughing through his nose and massaging his cysts with the Venus-less hand.

Charlie slumps against the wall like a macramé hanging, stands face-to-face with a bust of young Buddha. He tells Crazy Jeff about Cutting Day.

"Yer lazy ass missed a good one. Got the brother here to smoke a little Trainwreck."

"Enjoyable, right?" Crazy Jeff asks me.

"It . . . well . . . ," I smile, "sure fucked me up."

Jeff bows his head and laughs. Gloria shifts on the loveseat, drooling.

Next week, Crazy Jeff and Gloria are driving into Sacramento to protest "some new idiot proposition. I lose track of the numbers."

I run my fingers along the back of Johanna's neck, gather some of her hairline sweat as if essential nectar, the same stuff that stained our pillows in Chicago, the same stuff that, before my ass, stained so many others.

This numberless proposition that Crazy Jeff and Gloria despise seeks to regulate the ways in which medical marijuana will be distributed to patients, requiring them to reregister for government-issued identity cards.

"It's 848 all over again!" Crazy Jeff announces. "We already have ID cards! This would only make it harder to get them."

In 1999 Crazy Jeff and Gloria, along with many other medical marijuana patients, marched on the California capitol lawn to demonstrate against the infamous proposition.

"Gloria wore her 'Ban Aspirin!' T-shirt," Crazy Jeff says, turning his head and kissing the sleeping Gloria on her thigh. "We made it the night before with a black laundry marker. She was the talk, let me tell you. I have pictures!"

According to Crazy Jeff, Gloria was weak with illness during the Prop. 848 protest, riding a wheelchair into the committee meetings in her homemade T-shirt. One senator, championing the bill, gestured to the withdrawn Gloria as if she were evidence of the need for tighter regulation. He said something to the effect of, "Look at the type of people we're up against."

"Whereupon I said," Crazy Jeff declares, his head upturned to the Sofa Room's ceiling, "'Who? Sick people? People who this bill really affects?'"

He laughs, but this time, it's an angry laugh.

"Of course they shut me up," he continues, waving his arm up and down as if the Venus of Willendorf were reincarnated as a hammer. "The banging of the gavel, the leaning into the microphone . . . Very serious people."

"How's she doing now?" Johanna asks, gesturing to the dozing Gloria.

"Well, you know," Jeff shrugs, "it's all a roller coaster. Before you two arrived, she was feeling pretty bad, and had to use the wheelchair, but she was still out there picking. Of course, she didn't go up the slope. She had to stay at the bottom and in the greenhouse."

Jeff mimics the motion of a wheelchair rolling downhill and, wide-mouthed, captures the stunned face of its doomed rider. Then, the laughter, the cyst-rubbing.

"It's always gonna be a problem," Charlie contributes from his corner. He has, in fatigue, slumped a little further into the wall, as if the macramé were doused with a bucket of water. Still, he doesn't sit down.

Just to let you know: this dialogue, while not a perfect replica, is pretty damn close. Still, for the sake of consistency, consider me unreliable.

Proposition 848 specifically required that the California State Department of Health Services determine a rubric by which to judge a patient as either "qualified" or "unqualified" to receive an identity card and, therefore, medical marijuana. As such, the bill outlined a new set of "crimes" that could be tied into the issuances of these cards, any deviations punishable by law. Oftentimes, though, these "criminals" were those who used pot to staunch their puking up of bile. I'm sorry: was that too angry? I blame that blue wastebasket full of hair. I blame over a year's worth of fucking my wife silently, due to thin walls.

Champions of this bill wished to overturn the Compassionate Use Act of 1996, claiming that the act brought with it unforeseen problems that prevented law enforcement from doing their job.

"Yeah!" Crazy Jeff spews, the Venus threatening to burst the confines of his fist. "*Problems*! Like patients actually having access to their medicine."

Crazy Jeff argues that even if some of the product slipped through the cracks unregulated, the good outweighs the evil.

"For every kid shooting aspirin into a vein, half a million kids don't have a headache anymore!" Jeff cries, then laughs. "Ban aspirin! Ban aspirin!"

Gloria shifts on the couch. Charlie stretches in the corner. Lance is off somewhere doing Lance things, perhaps with Ruby. No doubt he is enjoying the warmer night, in one state of undress or another.

"We were all up in arms," Jeff says. "It was exhausting. After all the protesting, we needed *twice* as much medicine!"

Proposition 848 further claimed that there was no real way to measure pain; that there was no scientific way to determine if a suffering patient was or was not receiving adequate relief from conventional medicines; that more information was needed. Maybe the screams were the product of acting; the vomiting, of syrup of ipecac. Maybe chemotherapy really was just like the common cold, combatable with Vitamin C. Maybe sarcasm is, like my Jesus-freak brother-in-law assures me, the Devil's plaything, and I'm surely going to hell without sunscreen.

"And until they get that *information*, I'll keep taking the medicine that works best, thank you very much," Jeff says, miming the inhalation of an invisible joint.

Should this bill have been passed (it wasn't, thanks to the outspokenness of the Crazy Jeffs and Glorias of the world), no more than three employees could contribute to a medical marijuana harvest on a single grow site.

"So this would have benefited the black market pot dealers!" Crazy Jeff stresses.

"How so?" I ask.

"If cooperatives like Weckman were illegal, guess who would prosper? Patients could no longer cultivate their own medicine."

I picture Crazy Jeff and Gloria doggedly marching into one

fluorescent room after another, 1999 being a year of podiums and homemade T-shirts. Fluorescent lights and platters of their own butter cookies.

"And now, something similar is happening. The bastards would rather repeat history then learn from it."

"It's this bass-ackwards country," Charlie grumbles, the first time I'd heard *bass-ackwards* since high school chemistry class, when Mr. Ulrich (a champion bass fisherman during his summers off, coincidentally) used it to chastise Mike Sigal for lighting a Bunsen burner sans safety goggles.

"It's the whole world, really," Johanna says. "In Thailand you can get life imprisonment for selling pot. And did you know that even in the Bible, in Genesis, it says, 'God said, "Behold, I have given you every herb bearing seed which is upon the face of all the earth. To you it will be for meat."'"

Did I mention Johanna used to be a nun? In Key West, where we met waiting tables, she was known as Fallen Sister Johanna.

"Meat?" Charlie says. "Gimme mine mid-rare!"

"So what the hell?" Crazy Jeff asks. "Where does the problem come from?"

"Parasites and hypocrites," Charlie says, his voice scouring the air.

Throughout all of this political debate, the vetoes and the bills that pass, Crazy Jeff assures us, the harvest endures.

"When it comes right down to it," he says, "I believe that most of us at least don't want to be responsible for aggravating the agony of another."

"I do," Charlie says, smiling, "dependin' on who it is."

"You're an exception to most rules, Charlie," I say.

"Yep," he says, "I'm the exception."

Crazy Jeff repositions his head along Gloria's flank. She shifts and moans in her sleep. The plastic, wax, wooden icons of the Eastern religions look down on us from kitsch heaven, which may very well be the Sofa Room. Jeff tells us that, for Gloria especially, a little marijuana achieves what a mountain of prescription drugs could not.

"The conventional drugs are what fucked her up," Jeff says, "what fried her brain."

Perhaps this is the genesis of the rumors—of Gloria's falsely diagnosed paranoid schizophrenia.

"Until she rebounded a little bit, she had to be on the Boob Cocktail."

The Boob Cocktail Crazy Jeff refers to (also known at Weckman Farm as The Formula) is a tea of sorts made from soy milk with a marijuana infusion. The Formula is given to Patients who can not muster the strength to eat or smoke their medicine.

I watch Gloria's face. Her eyelids flutter as if crawling with ants, her left cheek beginning to spasm. Blessed be those who must take their medicine through a straw . . . Crazy Jeff tightens his grip on the Venus of Willendorf, this red ochre minigoddess blessing his hand with all things natural and voluptuous. I turn to Johanna and see that she is crying. I take her hand, kiss her knuckles. We are all tired. It's been a long day. I look forward to our tent, to our small space. But the whole of Weckman Farm has become a refuge, however wild—the sanctuary away from sanctuary. Whatever the fuck that means.

Gloria moans again in her sleep, and I envision my father lying in bed next to my mom, the red digitals of the alarm clock branding the room with the forthcoming day. I can tell he is awake by the way he holds his legs.

Gloria's moan increases in volume until she wakes herself up.

"Huh? Huh?" she murmurs, sitting up and staring, confounded, at all of us.

Crazy Jeff lifts his head from her hip. Gloria extends her fingers, meager as pencils. In waking, she is the anti-Venus, but a goddess nonetheless.

"Huuhhh," she says again, getting her bearings. "Well."

"You okay, honey?" Jeff asks.

"Something bad happened," Gloria says.

Collectively, I sense, our hearts shrink, our stomachs drop.

"What is it, baby?" Crazy Jeff says, brushing, with his fingertips, the hair from the corner of her mouth.

Johanna takes my hand. Gloria shakes her head. She looks warily around the room. For her, it seems, only Crazy Jeff is safe.

"C'mon," he says, "what's the matter?"

She lifts herself from orange pillows. She leans to Crazy Jeff's be-cysted ears. She whispers.

"I dreamed you died."

TONIGHT, we are superstitious. We gather at the door of Hector's giant tent. From inside, not even a snore. The air is cold, our breath frosting, tumbling over itself. Mine commingles with Johanna's, hers with Charlie's, his with Lance's and Ruby's. Ruby clings to Lance's arm, holding on for dear warmth, her meager Canned Heat concert T-shirt admitting Mendocino County's midnight air. This is Johanna's idea.

Clinging to Hector's tent door, the laminated photo of the now-weather-beaten Virgen de Guadalupe offers to us her carnations, her halo of gold foil. We mimic her down-turned eyes and say, together, a silent prayer for Gloria. On Weckman, we have to take what we can get, do what we can.

Even in her fevered sleep, her gaunt dreams, her monosyllabic utterances, Gloria exudes an abundance of what may only be illness. But in illness, she is robust. Like my mother, she exhibits a verve in her lethargy, because of her lethargy. We worry nonetheless. This is surely the verve of the soon-to-be-dead.

Lance chews a rope of Ruby's hair, grinds it in his teeth like sand until I swear I can hear it cracking. She has her hand under the back lip of his shirt but keeps it still, as stoic as the Venus of Willendorf bound in Crazy Jeff's grasp. Tonight, we are all busts of something— the hope of others forced upon us—but like all things plaster, wax, wood, impotent. But, boy, can we decorate a room. Sometimes, that's enough.

"It's cold," Ruby says to Lance, who says nothing.

Johanna presses against me. Charlie hugs himself, exhales through his nose. He is the first to say, "Amen."

A couple days ago, our supply bags were delivered, dropped off beneath the food tent by Lady Wanda's faceless, perhaps-elvish, messengers. As always, we searched among the paper bags for those labeled with our names. It was then that I learned of Charlie the Mechanic's love for dried papaya.

"Pure Hawaii," Charlie called it.

He takes a piece now from his pocket, this waxen orange cube, and holds it in his fingers, offering it to the Virgen. Then, pulling his arm at the shoulder, his right hand stretching behind his ear, Charlie throws the papaya into the air—this tropical centerfielder, this beautiful arc—skating across the moon, landing soundlessly in the crops, this sweet thing that came to Weckman from across the Pacific.

Charlie and his dead brother. Charlie and Vietnam. Charlie and the departing wife.

No one looks at Charlie. No one asks him why he did this.

Lance says, "Goodnight."

He and Ruby weave through the tents and disappear. Johanna and I turn for our Cimarron. I touch Charlie on the back.

"Hmm," Charlie says. "Least they have the unions."

"Yeah," I say.

Johanna kisses Charlie on the cheek.

Charlie is talking about the Medical Marijuana Patients Union (MMPU), who offer their support to activists like Crazy Jeff and Gloria. Since various counties in California are seeking to decimate the Compassionate Use Act via a cluster of proposed bills, the MMPU has intervened. Soliciting the aid of the American Civil Liberties Union (ACLU), the MMPU has insured that the affected patients receive proper legal representation.

These unions have a history of backing the likes of Crazy Jeff and Gloria. They routinely support other attacked organizations, including the Wo/Men's Alliance for Medical Marijuana (WAMM). Unlike Weckman Farm, which employs Patients and non-Patients alike,

WAMM is a collective of terminally ill Pickers and growers who have established a working hospice directly on the grow site.

In Sacramento, Crazy Jeff and Gloria are going to fight a proposition supporting federal law over state law. The advocates of this proposition argue that federal law, which bans the use of marijuana both medically and recreationally, trumps California's local policy. If this proposition successfully passes, WAMM, Lady Wanda, and many others (many of whom are combating illness) will have to uncover, if only for a short time, a different line of work.

Crazy Jeff said, back in the Sofa Room, that this would force Gloria to revisit "her garbage bags full of prescription drugs. The painkillers cause nausea, so she has to take an antinausea pill that causes headaches, so she has to take another one for that, which causes bladder infections . . . But we have a lot of friends."

"Yeah," Gloria followed, sitting up on the couch after her nap, her lower lip folded over her upper.

In addition to the ACLU, Crazy Jeff and Gloria's friends include the Americans for Safe Access (ASA), and the Drug Policy Alliance (colloquially known as The Alliance).

"And these are science people!" Jeff exclaimed. "Trust me. All of them have short hair."

"Yeah," Gloria said.

The ASA is indeed a collection of scientists, teachers, doctors, and patients hoping to provide safe and legal access to medical marijuana.

"And they've found," Jeff said, "that it reduces pain even in cancer patients and HIV/AIDS cases. And this way, we can avoid the addiction to the prescription shit. Gloria here . . ."

Crazy Jeff paused, swallowed, sighed.

"Gloria," he said.

"Huh?" she asked.

As of now, federal law does not acknowledge the scientific research Crazy Jeff so passionately cites. Federally, marijuana is classified as a Schedule One drug. This designation groups marijuana with drugs such as LSD and heroin; all Schedule One drugs are said, under federal law, to have no accepted medical use. As such, all research, completed or in progress, that counters this law is deemed unofficial. For years, the MMPU and its affiliates have been lobbying to reclassify marijuana, allowing the medical research federal recognition.

Extending its intimidation beyond its nickname, The Alliance argues that the real criminals are those who wish to overturn the Compassionate Use Act, robbing the ill of the medicine that works best and has among the least chances for dependency.

The proponents of these propositions believe that the Compassionate Use Act floats in the middle of a larger legal pool, in which California *criminal* law bans the use of marijuana under any condition. The new proposition inflaming the face of Crazy Jeff and sending Gloria deeper into the orange loveseat cushions wants to uphold these criminal laws, shunning even the identity card program as debated in the infamous Prop. 848.

"So now," Crazy Jeff continued while Gloria entered a sneezing fit, "they're saying the old ID cards and constant police checks of the IDs aren't enough. They want a total ban!"

Gloria wiped her nose and shook her head.

"Yeah," she said.

"And!" Crazy Jeff said. "Even with the federal law—The Prohibition! The Prohibition!—states have always been able to make their own program."

Gloria reached for his hand. He passed her the Venus of Willendorf and she held it to her face, as if a newspaper to nearsighted eyes.

"The fucked-up thing is," Crazy Jeff said, "is that it'll never pass. It's doomed from the start and I think they know it. But it takes so much energy to challenge it. They count on that. And we have to challenge it."

Backing the California MMPU and its national cohorts are attorneys general from Hawaii (good for both Charlie's papaya and medical marijuana), Oregon, and Colorado. The specific patients attacked in this new proposition (yes, names are mentioned) bear such burdens from sciatica to rectal cancer. Also targeted by name are the spouses and families of the patients, who administer, aid in, and/or bear witness to the usage of this controversial medicine, as well as the doctors who prescribed it, one of whom founded and manages a free HIV/AIDS clinic.

"Thank God they're helping us," Jeff said. "It's a big voice. Almost as loud as Gloria's. Whoo-hoo!"

"Whaaat?" Gloria said.

Crazy Jeff and Gloria are both members of the MMPU.

"Fifteen bucks a year dues," Jeff said. "Pretty tolerable."

"What do they do besides offer legal representation?" Johanna asked.

"Well!" Jeff chimed. "The legal stuff is a pretty big deal. Whoo-hoo-hoo! It's a big deal!"

I couldn't tell if his outbursts were genuine or facetious.

After calming down, Jeff discussed how the MMPU is like any other organization, prizing newsletters, community outreach, and education. The union works with teams of scientists, distributing medical findings to doctors and government officials, opening their membership doors to patients, caregivers, physicians, alternative healers, researchers, and the Lady Wandas of the world.

"You can probably get in now!" Crazy Jeff laughed, waving his hands to Johanna and me.

In recent years, the MMPU has become affiliated with (either officially or unofficially) the Multiple Sclerosis Society and AARP, among other organizations.

"So when I retire," Crazy Jeff cried, unable to stifle himself, "not only can I get a discount on a hotel room, I can . . . I can . . ."

But he was laughing too hard. Gloria blew her lower lip forward, the discharging of a demure, deflated gun.

Indeed, the union has numerous subdivisions, including a Seniors Union, a Multiple Sclerosis Patients Union, a Mental Health Patients Union, a Cancer Patients Union, a Gastro-Intestinal Patients Union, a Chronic Pain Union, and an HIV/AIDS Patients Union. Criminals all, huh?

In spite of the persistent actions of the MMPU and its subdivisions, the opposition proves just as tireless. Their many propositions include subdivisions of their own. In Sacramento, Crazy Jeff and Gloria will contend with such a subdivision, one demanding that the California Department of Health define a measured amount of marijuana that constitutes a two-month medical supply.

"What about the patient as an individual?!" Crazy Jeff complained.

Crazy Jeff's opponents (who he claims are "only concerned with a human being if they work in law enforcement") stress that, under the quagmire of current policy, the police have a difficult enough time knowing who and who not to arrest. Even under current California law, a medical marijuana patient can be legally arrested, but will likely escape conviction if he or she can prove (as the law refers to it) "medical need." For this notion as well, Crazy Jeff's opponents demand more information.

The new proposition seeks the conviction of a patient who possesses more than the politically defined two-month (or sixty-day) supply. And even if such propositions do not pass, Crazy Jeff, Gloria, and other patients can still be convicted under federal law, without the protection of the state.

"Federal raid! Federal raid! Leave us the fuck alone!" Crazy Jeff boomed, shaking his fists in the air, his back thumping Gloria's loveseat against the wall.

"Stop!" Gloria said.

We all turn to her, delighted at her public utterance of a new word.

"And how do you determine amount?" Crazy Jeff continued. "Are we talking about Trainwreck, Super Kush, or Mexican Regs?"

Jeff argued that marijuana's potency varies from strain to strain.

"If Gloria can't smoke, she can't eat," Jeff said with finality. "Plain and simple. She'd be nauseous all the time. I mean, when Gloria sees the sunrise, she throws up. If she sees a rabbit, she throws up. [I enjoyed, albeit morbidly, his examples here.] These propositions are death sentences for us . . . *if* they pass, which they won't. There are so many better things for us to be doing—on both sides of the issue—than *this*."

Charlie detached himself from the wall, sat on the floor. It was getting late.

When leaving the Sofa Room for the Residents' Camp, Crazy Jeff walked us to the door. Gloria watched us from the couch as if we were rare birds that she may not see again. Knysna Louries.

"I'll be happy if she makes it through the season," he said.

No laughing. His voice low, his cysts untouched.

"I've lost so many of my friends," he said.

When we hug him, he loses his craziness.

Unzipping our tent door, I turn and see Charlie, still fixed on the Virgen de Guadalupe. Johanna and I crawl in. We kiss. In it, sparks of Chicago, Key West, my old bedroom, my father's coughs, Johanna's family across an ocean; in it, all the heavy-handedness I can muster. We pull our lips apart, lie down on our respective sides, smell the canvas there. In the cold moon, flickering its light over the walls of our tent, I can picture Charlie's throwing arm, the tiny piece of papaya, downed in the pot fields, feeding so many ants.

Seven

DAYS LATER, we learn that Charlie the Mechanic's talent extends beyond his ability to hurl a piece of dried fruit.

Many seasonal workers on medical marijuana farms are not only social revolutionaries but artists, who, after garnering their substantial seasonal pay, take the rest of the year off to do, as Lady Wanda loves to put it, "what they were put on this earth to do." While this may be a generalization, it seems to be a popular one, confirmed by the Weckmanites who have worked various other farms.

For many pot farm workers, this means playing guitar or bass or drums in a coffeehouse or bar band. For others, this means making clay sculptures of humpback whales, their eyes made of dried English peas, the baleen constructed from old toothbrush bristles. (True: this was made by a Picker who, besides this one brief mention, will not be a character in this tale.) And for many others, this means acting in local theaters, singing and dancing and painting the backdrops.

At least once a season on Weckman Farm, the Residents' Camp launches an informal talent show. The temptation to go overboard in describing such a scene is fierce, and I will admit, up front, to some vicious forthcoming exaggeration, but all of it is nevertheless rooted in truth, albeit filtered through a plume of smoke and a susceptible brain.

Various instruments are trucked in from the home of one of Lady Wanda's friends, an ethnomusicologist living on the outskirts of

Mendocino. Should any of the Pickers be so inclined, they could borrow and play for a night such exotic instruments as the Japanese koto or the Zimbabwean *shona mbira*. This year, though, the instruments chosen are decidedly American: snare drums and trumpets and electric guitars.

Sculptors have the opportunity to talk about their work, singers to belt out their octaves, dancers to don their slippers, poets to bellow their verse. For this night, the carnival tents seem right at home; the only thing missing are the death-trap rides, the meth addicts who operate them, the clowns, and the corndogs. I don't think corndogs are part of Alex and Emily's repertoire.

Lady Wanda—tonight, a housefrocked roadie—sets up a small stage at the base of the crops, adorning it with speakers and multiple microphones, though the amplification is hardly necessary. We are, I suppose, miles from nowhere. I doubt even the longhorns the next ranch over would be able to hear us. She supplies us with a few stage lights and a few thin squares of colored plastic to slip over them, should we choose to bathe the crops in red or blue or green. She even brought in a crew to set everything up so we didn't have to miss a day in the fields. Joy. In these parts, Lady Wanda is friends with everybody.

We all gather on the lawn in front of the stage, Lance toward the front, craning his neck, Ruby beside him; Johanna sandwiched between Charlie and me. She keeps reaching forward and flicking Lance on the ear, Lance playing the seasonal role of her little brother.

"Enough!" he says, but Johanna is undeterred.

Soon, he turns around and bites her on the foot. We all roll to the ground, giggling, Charlie the Mechanic knocking into Crazy Jeff, who houses Gloria's head in his lap. I am playing a role I have never played—the freewheeling, almost-middle-aged, rolling on the grass, pot-smoking giggler, deserving of envy and scorn. I'm comfortable playing it here, until I think about it. Sometimes, self-awareness sucks.

"Orgy! Orgy!" Crazy Jeff cries, laughing, spittle flying wildly.

Shit. Am I becoming, in lifestyle, if not in looks, a pseudohippie? No. No. No. No.

Hector sits behind us and says nothing, just shakes his stationary head of hair at us. Bob, the ex-cop, is toward the back, his windbreaker swishing as he jogs in place, as if his turn onstage were the equivalent of a marathon.

I suppose I should just accept it: Weckman Farm has a way of reducing inhibitions. For weeks now, we have all been living on top of one another; eating, working, sleeping on top of one another. While this can stray toward the aggravating from time to time, the contained camaraderie of it all is rare and infectious. The farm encourages its crew to be more serious than usual, and sillier. It is in this quality—uninhibited and genuine—that Johanna and I take refuge. We are free to be scholars, and we are free to be idiots. At least this is what I tell myself. I'll spare you further talk—at least here—of cusps and cancer, of a weak comparison between a shifting life and plate tectonics, how frightening and depressing and fun it is to have once been some tragedy-free Pangaea, only to be blown apart into scattered crumbs of earth. (Cue violins, runny nose . . .)

Lance and Lady Wanda are set to take the stage first, she on vocals, he on guitar. On bass is one of the German Shepherd's Picker friends, a rail-thin ex–heroin addict named Billy the Painter. Rumor has it that Billy, both a house and fine art painter, came to Weckman to shake his hard-drug habit. Rumor also has it that Billy is a shit fetishist—in civilian life, he is known to don scuba gear and go swimming around in outhouse toilets. Charlie tells me that Billy was famous around San Francisco for his "scat parties."

Given the name, I don't press Charlie for details, but he continues, "I think it's just a buncha freaks sittin' in a circle, meditatin' around a big pile of shit."

This is one rumor I don't seek to confirm or dispel with Billy. I'm not precisely sure how to broach the subject, but I have, in my head, a lot of false starts. In the name of restraint, I'll keep them there.

A more benign rumor has it that Billy used to play in San Francisco's yearly Battle of the Bands competition, often reaching the finals against the then relatively unknown Dead Kennedys.

"And he always lost," Charlie makes sure I know.

Lance solicits me to play drums for them, a five-piece set that, while modest, injects my stomach with butterflies. I haven't played the drums for years. In high school, I was in a jazz fusion band called the Herky Jerky Movement, covering, badly, tunes by Chick Corea, the Weather Report, and other luminaries. This to popularity did not lead. But since then, I haven't played much. I decide to keep my role sololess and quiet, playing with brushes instead of sticks. Even so, I feel free to sound terrible.

An admission: My old jazz fusion band was actually called Cynosure, which sounded good enough in high school (and embodied, in definition, all the arrogance of a high schooler: *Something to which, due to its brilliance, all eyes are turned . . . Oooooo . . .*), but I now really like the name Herky Jerky Movement and often use this invented substitute when talking of my past at parties.

Billy takes the stage first. He is opening with the display of his latest painting, a four-by-three-foot canvas, the background painted a Bob's-windbreaker turquoise. In the middle of the foreground, a black design hovers, resembling the offspring of a scorpion and a cardboard box.

Whittled to the bone, even more so than Gloria, Billy raises the painting above his head. His elbows jut out like nickels. The sky is dark and starry; the stage is lit in a murky blue, the drum set staring my heart into abnormal palpitations.

"This is my new one," Billy crows to his audience of peers, his voice pitched high like a baby bird's.

The crowd hushes, considering Billy's work. Billy pauses and breathes heavily for an eternal sixty seconds, his nose upturned, perhaps seeking out the foulness of outhouse row.

Finally, he says, "Does anyone have any questions?"

"Do you exhibit anywhere?" one of the Pickers shouts, hidden among the seated crowd.

"At a few, well, a couple small galleries in San Fran," he chirps, offering no further elaboration.

He lowers his arms a bit, the bottom of the canvas resting on the crown of his head.

"What is it?" Bob asks.

Billy takes the canvas from his scalp and turns it to himself. He examines the work as if it were not his. He pauses again, considering.

"It's a Brain Freeze," he says.

Johanna looks to me, wrinkles her forehead.

"Shiiiit," Lance says.

Hector laughs dismissively through his teeth, passes a joint into the dark.

"Remember that movie *The Brain That Wouldn't Die?*" the German Shepherd calls from somewhere in the back.

No one answers, but Billy nods.

"I like it, Billy," the Shepherd approves. "It's very neurological."

"Thank you," Billy blushes.

Lady Wanda, waiting in the wings, steps forward.

"Time to pick up your bass, Billy," she says.

Johanna turns to me.

"Go," she says.

Lance and I stand simultaneously. He holds his fist to me, indicating that I should match his gesture. When I do, he touches his knuckles to mine. I feel I am back at summer camp, about to prove my weakness at kickball.

"All right . . ." he says.

Lady Wanda steps behind the microphone in a stunning midnight blue evening gown, her cleavage as deep as a well, inviting her audience to make a daunting wish; ample enough to house not only a few coins, but my entire bank account.

Lance hoists himself onto the stage, somersaulting and retrieving his acoustic guitar, now equipped with microphoned pickups. My ascent onto the stage is far less acrobatic—my back is sore from the fields—but my friends are clapping. Did I say *friends*?

"Bang them shits!" Charlie shouts.

I take this to mean something about my playing the drums.

In the blue light, I feel I am living in an aquarium, Lady Wanda the suckerfish about to ingest us all in the name of cleaning the tank.

I step toward the drum set, Billy the Painter pointing his bass at my chest like a bazooka. He is nodding and nodding, his eyes the fattest part of him.

Lance holds the face of his guitar toward me. During tonight's dinner, Lance handed me a piece of paper with the set list—a four-song foray into 1960s and 1970s folk rock.

"Real simple drumming," Lance said. "Nothing Brubeck."

I want to tell him Brubeck played piano, but I know what he means.

From the stage, I can see the plume of pot smoke resting over the crew. In the blue lights, it looks like the sky on Pluto. Here on Weckman Farm, it's still a planet. I lift the drum brushes from the snare and hold them over my head in an X. Idiot. Again, my friends clap. Hector grabs Johanna's shoulders and shakes her. Charlie emits a deafening whistle, his two pinky fingers anchored into the corners of his mouth. I don't think about my mom once.

Crazy Jeff screams, "Play it! Play it!" and wriggles with laughter.

From the stage, Weckman Farm looks huge: the crops tumbling over the hill and pooling at the bottom, the tent village approaching township incorporation, and behind us, the food tent, Lady Wanda's mansion, the curing shed, the tractors asleep like gorillas on their feet. And the colorful crew, quilting the grass, stoned and sober, tired and wide-awake.

Lady Wanda smacks me on the ass. Her eye shadow is green, her lipstick orange. Oddly enough, she looks beautiful, fully realized.

"Drum, honey," she urges, and I want to kiss her on the cleavage.

I mount the tattered red stool behind the set and spin nervously from left to right. Though only a five-piece set, the drums seem as complicated to navigate as an airplane control board. Billy wraps his fingers over the neck of the bass, Lance spins in a circle, wearing his guitar high on his chest. Lady Wanda leans salaciously into the microphone, the stand perfectly flanked by her breasts. I apologize for this obsession, but you should've seen 'em that night!

"On 'Wideband' everybody!" Lance calls to us, referencing his countdown alternative to 1-2-3.

I tighten my grip on the drum brushes, squint through the blue to see Johanna's smiling face.

"Coaxial! Tubular! Wideband!"

In a pop of sound, all instruments ignite, Lady Wanda crooning a mouthful of "Oooooooos" into the microphone.

I fall into the rhythm easily. The song is simple, Barry McGuire's "Eve of Destruction," Lady Wanda transcending McGuire's rasp, reaching somewhere between Nina Simone and opera.

Lance, a miniature Pete Townshend, waves his strumming arm in a circle, windmilling the strings. Billy stands almost perfectly still, his emaciated fingers dancing, strings meeting strings. Occasionally, he bends his knees, then straightens. This, for Billy, seems an act of God.

Lady Wanda sings:

You don't believe in war,
but what's that gun you're totin'
And even the Jordan River
has bodies floatin'

Charlie bellows, "Yeeeeaaaahhh!"

Hector follows suit, pumping his fist in the air. Ruby stands to the side of the stage in a long skirt, whirling like a Sufi dervish.

Lady Wanda bends further to the microphone, lending a carnal element to protest. She points to the crowd, and even from my perch behind the drums, I can see that her fingernails are painted black. If I were seventeen, I would've had a wicked boner. She raises her voice.

As if on cue, the crew roars. Johanna is now up and swaying with Ruby (something heretofore unexpected and out of character for her); Hector stands behind them, looking at me and making rabbit-ears with his fingers behind their heads. I want to hug him, hard and for a long time.

I lean into the cymbal, tickling it with the brushes, stirring a sound like wind through a tunnel. Lady Wanda reaches toward the crew like a healing televangelist and begins the second verse.

As the song crescendos, then ends, Lance flailing his head as if it were on fire, we're acknowledged with cheers. I must admit, it feels good to drum again; reminds me of a time when Chicago was my home, my parents young and healthy. (Insert your own rendition of "Carefree Highway" here.) Johanna blows me a kiss.

We make our way through three more songs: Ramblin' Jack Elliott's "San Francisco Bay Blues," a pianoless version of Janice Joplin's "Half Moon" (Lady Wanda hamming it up, prowling the stage like a butterfly hunter), and Bob Dylan's "Idiot Wind" (Lady Wanda and Lance singing the chorus together, sharing the microphone).

Our set complete, I jump from the drum stool, stand in line with Billy, Lance, and Lady Wanda, and bow. Lance turns to me.

"Not bad, man," he says.

I shrug. Billy puts his fists together and raises each pinky, making a set of devil's horns.

"Metal," Billy says. "Metal."

Lady Wanda kisses me on the lips, smearing my face with orange. In her neck, I smell lavender. I fold into her like an extra pinch of flour into bread dough. I don't want her to let go of me, but when she does, I feel anointed.

"Thank you," I say.

"Honey, please," she says.

We rejoin the crew on the lawn, Lady Wanda standing to the side of the stage, acting as emcee.

Johanna hugs me, kisses me, Ruby hugs Lance, kisses Lance, a few Pickers pat Billy on the back, and Charlie stands.

"Nice, brother," he says to me.

"Nice, brother," he says to Lance.

"Charlie, it's you," Lady Wanda says.

"Where is it?" Charlie calls into the blue stage lights.

"Right here," Lady Wanda says, producing a burnished trumpet from behind the stage. "Mother-of-pearl keys, like you asked for, honey."

"Didn't think ya'd get it," he says, dismissively and unimpressed.

"Trumpet?" I ask Charlie as he starts for the stage.

"Yep," he says. "Gotta make some noise."

BILLY BACKS UP Charlie on bass. Even so fragile, Billy looks like he can do this forever. Someone passes me a joint and I take what I tell myself is my last drag of the evening. I'm feeling it. Charlie walks to center stage, bathed in blue light, smoke from our polluted exhales. He raises the trumpet's mouthpiece to his lips like a martini glass, an ex-alcoholic about to take his first sip in years. For his sake, I hope the olives are stuffed with blue cheese. I have no idea what that means.

Lance turns, tells us, "This is his own composition."

No *shit*, I think and, maybe, say.

Charlie plays. He plays, his cheeks inflated, his fingers reeling. He plays with his eyes closed, surely envisioning countless firebombings and the scotches and water that took them away. We all fall silent and slack-mouthed. Johanna can only touch my knee. I can only breathe. Even the lit joints rest forgotten between the crew's fingers, frozen in time. The crops arc toward us, jealous of our heat. Our smoke is the only thing moving.

He plays soft, clean, a bar of Dove soap in the mouth of a baby. His lungs battle with a lifetime of inhalants—cigarettes, napalm, Trainwreck. Partnered with a trumpet, his lungs win by a mile. This is miracle and miracle and miracle.

Of the Residents' Camp, Charlie makes a nightclub. Billy supersedes his fetishes, becomes almost classy. Leaning into his bass, he could be wearing a tuxedo and a shimmering tie. His blonde hair would not be escaping from his ponytail, if only for this night, the wayward strands smoothed in slickness beneath a navy fedora.

And Charlie, a conductor: commanding Bob to touch the place of his zipped-up windbreaker under which lies his heart; Lance's capacity for love exploding like a water balloon, Ruby's long hair coming to dead rest on his thigh; Crazy Jeff and Gloria ready to overthrow the government and the heavy pages of heartless proposals;

Hector ready to climb from his treetop perch unafraid, descend into a Chiapas trova bar, his rifle replaced by a sweating bottle of Leon Negra; Waldo, found.

In this, Hector can fill his big tent with something bigger. Even the German Shepherd removes his wine coaster glasses, touches the earpiece to his lips as if he himself is about to play something visionary. The stethoscope, curled into his duck-hunter's coat, only wants to unravel, to turn its microphone to the music. Lady Wanda snakes an arm beneath her breasts, holds them up, as if this is the one way she can offer her heart to Charlie's song. The sequins on her gown catch thousands of tiny moons, competing bursts of light. This is a music during which infants become adults and adults become old. This is a music that allows age to become the name of a dance.

Johanna's mouth seizes.

She pronounces, "G— . . ." certainly about to say "God," but arrested by a trumpet, and all things unpronounceable.

Charlie receives the power of Lady Wanda's THE MEANING OF WORK handbook and transforms it into song—the Hebrew mystics and Irish folklorists joining hands somewhere in the nebula, swaying like ribbons, just slightly stoned on music and the cloud that rises from the crew.

Tonight, Weckman Farm achieves a new kind of exoticism. This is our underground club in Paris, lit blue as ice, the air crisp as a lime, and as penetrating. Our breaths and their passengers—carbon dioxide and marijuana—couple to produce a warmer air, even as the lawn cools. Charlie never opens his eyes. Never raises or lowers his instrument, but stands, a statue, this fountain of Mercury spitting the loveliest of waters.

He wails into the thing, a wail at once intense and soft as carpet, a night train from a mile away, the sleeper cars rattling. When speaking through the instrument, Charlie's voice is no longer electric; only in this way can he give us a lullaby. I squint in the blue haze, swimming. Looking down, I notice that Charlie has changed his shoes; instead of his work shoes—a filthy pair of off-white high-tops, he wears onstage black polished loafers, catching the light of Lady Wanda's dress. *Where the fuck did he get those?* If I wasn't so taken, I would have said to Johanna something smart-ass about him over-watching *The Shawshank Redemption*, but I didn't.

Somehow, perhaps in the trumpet's staccato, the wind around us stutters, vibrates, skips a few frames. Charlie must be taming the weather, charming this Mendocino cobra into submission. The sound sheers above us, a meat cleaver chopping the air into cookable pieces. Lady Wanda's hair whips upward. When a synthetic white light appears in the sky next to the moon, she raises her breasts even higher. Charlie never opens his eyes.

The helicopter sweeps over the crops, its searchlight waving over the plants, the California Department of Justice officials out of earshot of the show. I grasp Johanna's hand, my babbling heart running in circles with its head cut off. Only on Weckman Farm could imminent doom have such a gorgeous score.

In these flying searchlights, I see neighboring prison cells, Johanna and I kissing through a sliver in the cinderblock, just wide enough for our tongues. I see my father bringing us care packages—decks of cards and paperback bestsellers, trail mix and beef jerky, pomegranate-flavored water and wasabi peas. We must hear of my mother's condition during visitor's hours.

When the helicopter dips, Charlie continues to dazzle onstage. I can't picture him behind bars. Hasn't he been through enough? And Lance and Ruby having just discovered each other! Alex, Emily, and Antonio forced to survive on prison food? And Hector, so used to the space of his tent and the quietness of his tree. And Bob, so eager to make friends, he's willing to make enemies. And Crazy Jeff and Gloria, having so many protests ahead of them, so much healing to do. And Lady Wanda in her evening gown, this blue sequined billboard of festivity; surely they'd let her change before taking her in . . .

This is the first real intrusion on Weckman Farm since we've been here, and never has the outside world seemed so harsh, dangerous, and foreign. Not until the Department of Justice's searchlight crosses the crew do I realize how safe we've felt here—on a farm that skirts legality.

And now the monster in the closet has thrown off our blankets, and all we can do is face it, stare its light back into hiding with the only weapon we have: a Vietnam vet with brass in his mouth.

And Charlie plays, the trumpet calling to its siblings: every instrument blown and plucked, pounded and strummed, every wand, every wizard's crooked staff. The notes spill over one another, a twenty-car pileup in D-minor, a cauldron bubbling with spells. The searchlight traces from the crops to the crew to the tent village, lawful fear in the bright mask of something holy. We hold our collective breath and allow Charlie to resuscitate.

After hovering for what must only be a couple minutes, the helicopter shoots away from Weckman, flies in the direction of the longhorn ranch and cemetery. If Lady Wanda is growing more plants than she has a permit for, Charlie's trumpet enacts a cosmic sleight of hand, the extra offenders disappearing into a world of illicit smoke and mirrors. Billy, shielded behind his bass, watches the helicopter fade into the distance, on its nocturnal rounds.

So thin, Billy shudders as if touched by a ghost. Oblivious, or pretending to be, Charlie hits a note on the high end of the scale, toying with the dead ends of frequency, then follows with one so low we can barely hear it. The earth itself begins to hum. The core spits like oatmeal. He holds the note for twenty seconds, his red face, coupled with the blue light, going purple. His face full of blood, Charlie takes the instrument from his mouth. In this small silence, the insects assert themselves, whooshing in their nighttime flight and ritual. Tonight, we win.

CHARLIE PLAYS THIS unbroken song for twenty-two minutes and stops. We all throw in our pennies but have already received our wish. To the applause, Charlie dips the trumpet; the instrument does the bowing for him. He leans into the microphone.

"Ya'll see that helicopter?" he asks.

The crew, in unison, sighs, "Whew."

Lady Wanda mutters, "Can't believe Johnny Screw's up this late."

Charlie steps from the stage, his posture a little straighter than before. I never thought I'd call Charlie the Mechanic *graceful*.

Behind us, I hear the Shepherd say, "The trumpet fought the law and the trumpet won. Unprecedented!"

Lady Wanda embraces Charlie, points to the sky, and whispers something in his ear. Charlie laughs. I want to know, but will not ask him. He hands the instrument to her and cracks his knuckles, raises his hands over his head, fingers still netted together in encomium to the night and the forthcoming morning that carries with it, assured fatigue. His posture is so perfect, I wish Robbi were here (instead of with her giant seasonal Fort Bragg boyfriend) to offer a yoga analysis of Charlie's moon salutation. He lowers his hands and rejoins his place on the lawn. I look at him and shake my head.

"Unbelievable," I say. "I had no idea . . ."

"I know," Charlie says. "Those bastards coulda raided us."

"No, I mean . . ."

"Coulda *raided* us," Charlie stresses.

Again, Johanna says, "G— . . ."

AFTER CHARLIE'S SET, the Residents' Camp Talent Show descends into a mishmash of pottery; homemade jewelry; poetry readings flamboyant and demure; Masonite carvings of severed body parts, printed and captioned with such antinuclear war slogans as "Don't Let the Portabella Get Ya!"; Act One, Scene One of *How to Succeed in Business Without Really Trying* performed as a puppet show, Finch made of twigs and dried flowers, Bud Frump made of tin cans and shoelaces.

The rest of my friends remain in the crowd, never taking the stage. Alex, Emily, and Antonio sit in the back, preparing for their breakfast-time talent show beneath the food tent. Approaching two thirty in the morning, Lady Wanda steps again to the microphone.

"'Idiot Wind,'" Bob shouts. "Encore!"

Lady Wanda laughs, but she looks ready to get out of that dress.

"Great job as always, everyone," she says. "We'll talk tomorrow about our little visitors. Get some sleep. Tomorrow, we start late. Ten o'clock."

The crew cheers louder than they did for Charlie.

Eight

WAS THAT HELICOPTER really flown by the California Department of Justice? I don't know, and of course . . . As a result of incidents like last night's and other motivations—justified, unjustified, ill-defined, and precise—Lady Wanda has been employing snipers at Weckman Farm since 1997. (I must pat myself on the back for meticulously wording my questions to her so as not to appear like an interviewer, though this self-congratulation, upon examination, is for nothing more than my ability to deceive a trusting person. Now I feel bad about myself, and revoke said pat.) Though an avid gun collector herself (her antique gun collection includes such weaponry as an 1865 Belgian cavalry snap hook and an 1891 Argentinean navy nickel-plated rifle—both fully badass), she used to be against having firearms on Weckman, believing their presence would provoke violence. After the passing of the Compassionate Use Act in 1996, Lady Wanda was the victim of a governmental and grassroots backlash. And not *that* grass. Ho, ho.

During 1996's harvest, Weckman Farm was twice invaded illegally: once by CAMP, California's Campaign Against Marijuana Planting, a division of the Department of Justice and Bureau of Narcotic Enforcement; once by a private vigilante militia, whose guns were neither Belgian nor Argentinean, were not from the nineteenth century, and were not safely locked behind Lucite. According to Lady Wanda, these private militias are increasing in number, staging armed raids on numerous marijuana farms both commercial and medical.

Over breakfast on our late-starting workday, the crew still digesting the last notes of Charlie's trumpet song, Lady Wanda tells us, "Those were CAMP officials in that helicopter last night."

I'm not sure how she knows this—the color of the copter, the style of flying? Did the starlight reflecting from her bosom illuminate their faces?

After last night's evening gown, Lady Wanda has returned to her trusty housefrock—this one bearing carnations not unlike those adorning Hector's Virgen de Guadalupe.

"They usually leave us alone," she says.

During the talent show, it was Waldo, Hector's epileptic replacement in sniperdom, who was stationed in the redwood tree. I could only speculate on his internal debate about whether to fire, like the hero of so many Schwarzenegger movies, into the blades of the CAMP helicopter, spawning a midair explosion and the rock 'n' roll–fueled progression of Weckman Farm's end credits.

Lady Wanda tells us that CAMP typically concentrates its efforts on commercial, nonmedical marijuana farms, but the agency has been known to stage raids without such discrimination. In 2004 alone, CAMP is said (by Lady Wanda) to have destroyed over one million marijuana plants on farms both commercial and medical. While these raids of medical marijuana farms are considered illegal within the parameters of the Compassionate Use Act, they are legitimate on the federal level, and allowed to go on without repercussion. (Unless maiming and killing still keep people up at night.)

The number of plants confiscated during the Northern California marijuana harvest has increased from approximately 350,000 in 2001 to 1,700,000 in 2006. This can speak either to the stepped-up efforts of CAMP and other law enforcement, or to the increase in regional pot production.

"Either way, no one protects us," Lady Wanda says, last night's green eye shadow still clinging, faded, to her lids. Johanna and I look at each other, both of us (I'm guessing) contemplating the nature of *protection*—its contexts.

CAMP was founded in 1983 and is made up of agencies at local, state, and federal levels. It remains the largest legislative enforcement task force in the United States, incorporating divisions of the California National Guard, the California Department of Fish and Game, the federal DEA, the Bureau of Land Management, the U.S. Forest Service, the MET (Marijuana Eradication Team), COMMET (County of Mendocino Marijuana Eradication Team), and countless local police departments. (This is the acronym section of the book, or ASB.) CAMP has divided itself into five groups, each responsible for patrolling a specific region within California.

Many speculate (Lady Wanda among them) that the Reagan administration created CAMP to prove to South American governments that the United States does not tolerate the cultivation of any illegal drug; as such, these foreign governments were urged to adopt a policy of zero tolerance as well. Pardon me while I clear my throat of the peppercorn of unrealistic expectations.

Numerous stories circulate throughout Mendocino County's medical marijuana farms about the lawless CAMP "warriors," as Lady Wanda calls them, storming property, indiscriminately destroying crops, beating crew members, cutting irrigation hoses, slaughtering farm dogs, and spawning the occasional shootout. In turn, marijuana prices skyrocketed because of the risk.

According to Lady Wanda, the CAMP officials meet before a raid, staging a "frat boy pep rally." Often donning military camouflage gear, AK-47s, and M-16s, the Short-Term Airborne Operations division of CAMP boards their helicopters and flies low over a series of marijuana farms. Sometimes, a team will land, releasing a be-gunned, government-sanctioned army into the fields.

CAMP claims to gather information on the "legality" of these farms either from local county officials or from impromptu flyovers and visual assessments. Armed with detailed maps, the officials in a CAMP helicopter will sometimes hover over a crop (as they did last night), counting from the air the individual plants. If, from this perspective, they believe the crop to be in excess of the permitted amount, they will often land.

"If they land," Lady Wanda says, "watch out."

I look at Johanna.

"What have we gotten into?" I ask, hoping our story doesn't become some political thriller of the fields. *If you smoke it, they will come . . .*

Lance tells us, over yet another granola and plain yogurt breakfast (what Johanna has begun referring to as "Blowgurt"), that when he was still a teenage Picker at Weckman, a CAMP official broke his arm before leading a raid on the crop.

"Not a surprise," Charlie says.

Ruby slides closer to Lance.

"Did it hurt?" she asks.

"Uh . . . yeah," Lance says.

CAMP commanders routinely claim that "to their knowledge" they have not been involved in a medical marijuana raid since the passing of the Compassionate Use Act. Lady Wanda, a victim of such raids, dismisses this claim with a wave of her black-fingernailed hand.

"Sometimes they raid by car," she says, "with dogs."

The dogs in these cases, she says, are violent animals who chase down any crew member who dares to flee. CAMP claims that these dogs are a necessary protective measure since many marijuana farms operate with armed guards. Again, the complicated nature of protection asserts itself into the air between Johanna and me, making for a thoughtful, if confusing, ménage a trois. If a CAMP team raids a marijuana farm, medical or otherwise, shootouts are not uncommon. Both CAMP officials and cultivators have been killed in gunfire exchanges.

"A lot of medical marijuana farms are antiweapon," Lady Wanda says. "I used to be, too."

After these violent raids, Lady Wanda began to employ snipers.

"If only to put a stop to these hell hounds," she says. "Otherwise, we'll get torn to pieces."

Certain farms in the area have joined to launch an insurance fund that would cover, at least in part, the financial losses caused by such raids.

When raiding by road vehicle, CAMP officials will sometimes park at a distance, leap from the back of a large truck, their weaponry clattering against their hips, and crest a series of rolling slopes. (Allow me a few liberties here for dramatic effect.) From this vantage point, the eyes can assess the crop without the distraction of a vibrating helicopter engine. The CAMP officials will compare their estimates.

"And if they decide to raid," Lady Wanda says, "it's gonna look like *Braveheart* for a little while."

Lady Wanda tells us of a CAMP raid during which her entire crop was confiscated. Additionally, the officers stole a large sum of money, broke Lance's arm, and shot two Pickers, wounding them.

"And if you think a dog biting someone in the ass is funny, you shoulda seen it that year," Lady Wanda says, "when they ripped chunks of this guy's muscle right out. He was an AIDS patient, trying to get away. But he couldn't run fast enough."

As if Weckman Farm wasn't interesting enough already, I try to imagine the property strewn with an excised gluteus maximus.

After particularly violent raids, many growers and their crews will abandon a farm, leaving behind that atmosphere of my often-imagined "lost colony." Sometimes, all that remain are discarded skillets and abandoned tents. As Lady Wanda addresses us, granola and sour yogurt revolving around my mouth, I pray my paranoid visions are not prophetic.

Not all CAMP raids result in violence; many simply involve the confiscation of the crop and the arresting and deportation of illegal immigrants, but as Lady Wanda says, "You can never tell with people."

CAMP officials claim that many marijuana farms in California are owned by Mexican drug cartels. On the federal level, the DEA supports this claim, further speculating that various Asian mafias own many of California's medical marijuana dispensaries and hospices.

Lady Wanda dismisses these claims with the violent shaking of her arms. Her black fingernails dig into the meat of her palms, her fists raised above her head as if firing two invisible machine guns into the air.

"Preposterous!" she says. "This has become a billion-dollar publicity stunt that costs lives!"

While she admits that certain "underhanded groups are known to contribute to this industry," the blanket accusations made by CAMP and the DEA aim to divert public support and local legislators away from the marijuana farms, medical or otherwise.

"These tabloid allegations," Lady Wanda says, "are the only way they can justify this violence to the public."

Crazy Jeff, uncharacteristically devouring his granola, puts down his spoon and begins clapping his hands.

"This is what happens when self-righteousness justifies violence," Crazy Jeff tells our table of regulars.

"Whole fuckin' world, brother," Charlie says, reaching across the table and touching knuckles with Johanna.

"Civil rights my ass!" Crazy Jeff says. "It's a dinosaur! It's a dinosaur!"

"Tyrannosaurus Rex!" Bob contributes, his windbreaker swishing as he raises his arms, looking around for any form of acceptance. I wink at him and this seems to satisfy.

Lady Wanda tells us that CAMP further justifies its actions in environmental terms. Indeed, in California, many commercial marijuana farms are less environmentally sensitive than the medical ones. CAMP rightfully stresses that these farms utilize harmful nitrogen fertilizers, pesticides like malathion, and rat poison; the crew members litter the countryside with their trash; the outdoor restroom facilities permeate the local water supply.

But Lady Wanda argues that CAMP occasionally disregards these discrepancies between commercial farms and many medical marijuana farms in favor of indiscriminate raiding.

"And besides," she says, "how many gallons of fuel do you think these helicopters burn per day?"

Again, Crazy Jeff claps. Gloria throws her head backward, but I don't think it's intentional. Lance and Ruby hold hands. I listen for some oddly literate interjection from the German Shepherd, but there is none.

Many residents in these rural areas also argue that the helicopters are a local nuisance and source of noise pollution. As such, certain California county boards have launched campaigns against CAMP and its methods; local officials have run for office on tickets promising to control the organization.

Further, local advocate groups for the legalization of marijuana have asked CAMP whether legal cultivation would eradicate some of the alleged environmental damage. CAMP believes it would not, claiming that the issue of legalizing marijuana is too low on the priority lists of the local governments to be realistic, and stressing that marijuana remains a gateway drug for methamphetamine, cocaine, and heroin.

Lady Wanda shakes her fists in the air again.

"How many of you came here to *kick* hard drugs?" she asks the crew.

Mouths full of granola, a number of Pickers emit a low murmur.

In Lady Wanda's experience, marijuana is more of a gateway to sobriety than anything else. She argues that the funding given to CAMP should be diverted to a task force launched to control the thriving crystal-meth lab industry.

A local law enforcement official associated with CAMP recently equated the "war on marijuana" with the fight against rape, homicide, and drunk driving. Lady Wanda and Crazy Jeff groan, fueling each other's outrage.

"Smoking marijuana is not like drunk driving!" Crazy Jeff yells. "Driving stoned is like drunk driving!"

"Yep," Charlie says.

"And rape and murder?" Jeff continues. "That's like saying taking a prescription painkiller is the same as rape and murder! Where do these people come from? We have to promote education! The unions . . ."

"Well, for now, Jeff," Lady Wanda interrupts, "we are still forced to be mysterious."

Crazy Jeff sighs and Gloria sighs next to him, and I sigh now with mixed feelings as I write about this life.

Lady Wanda continues to talk about the 1996 raids on Weckman Farm. The real violent danger, she says, comes not from CAMP, but from heavily armed and unregulated anti-marijuana vigilante groups. Even from these militia-style groups, the government and local law enforcement offer the Lady Wandas of the world no protection, no matter the context; often, they dismiss the resulting "massacres" (Lady Wanda's word) as par for the course.

"You play with fire . . ." Lady Wanda says, imitating a local sheriff. The more I hear, the more I am thankful for Charlie's trumpet.

FALL 1996, Lady Wanda sat on her veranda sipping from a cup of coffee with too much sugar. The weather was still tolerant of her penchant for housefrocks—maybe the one she was wearing was the solid pink with holes at the elbows, or the newer-looking one bespattered with daisies.

This must have been before Lance's time at the farm, though Lady Wanda speaks of him as if he's always been there, leading her crew. He would have only been thirteen at the time. I wonder what he was doing when he was thirteen. I wonder where he was. None of the present-day crewmembers would have been there. But Lady Wanda was there, likely supervising a much smaller crew.

I wonder if we all had our 1996 *equivalents*, to use Hector's favorite word. Surely, Lance had a counterpart, another young, beautiful man leading the picking crew with hair permanently convertible-whipped. Certainly, there would have been 1996 versions of Crazy Jeff and Gloria, activist Patients educating the newbies on a series of *-tion* words: legislation, frustration, medication . . . Bob, of course, is timeless; there's one of him in every city in the world. A crew of Bobs could have populated Weckman Farm in 1996. I wonder if Lady Wanda employed a house doctor back then. I wonder if Charlie the Mechanic, even in imagination only, is replicable. I wonder which young couple in 1996 stupidly felt they could escape a parent's mortality by fleeing here. All I know is that in 1996, Weckman Farm was sniperless.

Though the air was still warm enough for housefrocks, it would have been cool enough to drop the temperature of Lady Wanda's coffee.

"I remember I was stirring it with my finger," she says.

I imagine her pinky finger, the nail painted black, dipping beneath the surface of her coffee, whisking the sugar granules into dissolving. The Pickers would have been in the fields, arms thrust deep into the plants, the sticky residue inflaming their bodies in itch and stench. In 1996 Lady Wanda had only one chef working for her.

"Not nearly as talented as who you all have cooking for you," she says.

I imagine sodden scrambled eggs, bloated in a steam tray, losing their heat; horrible white bread still in the twist-tied plastic bag; margarine packets. This was the food driving the picking crew as Lady Wanda sipped her coffee and perhaps made a few phone calls to local dispensaries.

"Commercial farms have always had armed guards," Lady Wanda says. "But as I said, many of the medical marijuana farms shunned the presence of firearms. Many still do. But our neighbors, the people living around here for years, they've gotten to know where the medical marijuana farms are."

In the past, these "neighbors" have crashed the marijuana farms in two popular forms: sometimes in the guise of an anti-marijuana militia, sometimes as gun-toting potheads looking for a free score.

"Either way, we're robbed," Lady Wanda says.

As she finished her coffee, the undissolved sugar sludge coppered at the cup's bottom, Lady Wanda noticed four people in the distance, wearing camouflage gear and dark baseball caps. They were running across the property, across the stretch of lawn in between the present-day food tent and Residents' Camp, toward the crop fields. By the way they were holding their arms, she could tell that their guns were already in their hands.

The equivalent of Charlie the Mechanic would have been carrying a crate of marijuana buds to his one-seat tractor. In response to a comment shouted from another row (a "field holler," as it's become known on Weckman), the Charlie equivalent would have called, "That's it, brother!"

As he stepped from his row into Tractor Alley, the first of the militia would have shot him in the chest. In the fields, heads turning, scissors dropping. A strong man, the equivalent of Charlie the Mechanic would have held onto his crate even as he bled, the lawn cooling his back, the winds ruffling his sandy hair. In the clouds, he would have seen a massive bird turn into an airplane, a vision that would take him back to Vietnam. He would think of his wife as the second of the militiamen stepped toward him and, with heavy boots, kicked the crate from his hands. A constellation of Trainwreck or Durban Poison or Grand Daddy Purple would have erupted to the sky, a few falling into the tangle of Charlie's hair. Is this too much? Too melodramatic? Maybe. But if this work is nonfiction, I'm representing my wistful mood. Trying to, however unreliably. Anyhow, it's almost over.

The militiamen would have moved on, shooting eight Pickers, sending the rest of the crew scattering uphill and down, running toward the longhorn range, running toward the cemetery. (Wow. I didn't even intend those implications.) Then, the militia set about burning a segment of the crop. As the first tendrils of smoke kicked into the air like waterspouts, Lady Wanda paced the veranda, grasping her empty coffee cup by its handle.

"You're in shock," she says. "You don't know what to do. I mean, this happened all the time. It still happens all the time, but you just hear about it happening on other farms, to other growers and crews."

These militias, through their own networks and grapevines, garner maps of the marijuana farms in a certain region and proceed to strong-arm the growers and crew, oftentimes demanding a payoff.

"I called the local cops," Lady Wanda says. "I had to. They were shooting my crew. But there's always the risk of the local cops ratting you out, handing you over to the feds."

Again, I look to Johanna. I feel nervous and cinematic. For the first time in our lives, we are in a place where the word *feds* is used daily.

The equivalents of Crazy Jeff and Gloria got away unshot. The militiamen didn't have the time to hunt everyone down. They never do. Luckily, they didn't hit any Patients. The Bob equivalent was shot in the shoulder, bleeding under his windbreaker; the Lance was shot through the hand while running, shielding himself in whatever way possible. The 1996 version of Charlie the Mechanic was the only one who died. He never got to play his trumpet. The rest had their wounds treated in the small local hospital, the bills likely unpaid to this day.

"And the fuckers were never caught," Lady Wanda says, our breakfast granola frozen in our bowls. "They never are."

After shooting the crew and burning half of Lady Wanda's crop, the militiamen escaped into the woods before the police arrived.

"Unless one of these militiamen shoots a cop, the cops never go after them. I mean, who are we? It's just another pot farm shooting. We were just lucky we weren't turned in," Lady Wanda says.

Johanna takes my hand, pins it to the picnic bench. The real Charlie shakes his head, lays his hands flat on the rust-painted picnic table. I stare at his face so long I can see the pores in his cheeks, the tiny stubble that's beginning to poke from them. He has razor burn beneath his chin. The wind has blown a tiny white crumb of something into his left eyebrow. I am thankful he is here, breathing, his blood inside him. I say it quietly to myself, as if in first grade in November: *I am thankful for Charlie.*

Lance looks at his lap, Ruby running her unpainted, bitten fingernails over his back. His hands are filthy but perfect, held together with twenty-four-year-old skin. He's biting his lip, his eyes glazed over as if envisioning this 1996 invasion when he was barely into his teens; as if he had been there. From his mouth, there is no "Shiiiiiiit."

Bob is quiet, his windbreaker holding back its swish. Crazy Jeff rubs his cysts, but there is no laughter to stifle. Gloria scratches her neck. Hector is somewhere up in the redwood trees, watching for another attack.

The year following the militiaman invasion, Lady Wanda employed her first team of snipers.

These attacks happen every year, multiple times a year; much of the time, these incidents are not reported.

"Unless law enforcement is shot," Lady Wanda says. "Then it's all over the news and the fingers point to us. And we're peaceful people! But still, the legislators begin making their propositions and the clusterfuck starts all over again."

Last year, when local police were raiding a farm not too far from Weckman, a young man crested a hillside and opened fire. A shootout ensued, but the young man escaped; no one was injured. Earlier that year, a deputy in another county was shot and killed while raiding a marijuana farm. Again, the shooter escaped.

Mendocino County police have begun using infrared spotting helicopters to locate fleeing suspects at night. Because of the heat, when staging raids on marijuana farms, many authorities in Mendocino and neighboring counties (Sonoma, Lake, Humboldt) do not wear body armor. Since these raids often entail a great deal of trail-less hiking, the body armor is too much weight to bear, especially when one is carrying guns, machetes, and canteens of water.

Acts of violence on marijuana farms have become so common that the locals refer to early incidents as "the opening shots of the season." Growers are shot to death by their crew members; crew members suspected of robbery are shot to death by their bosses; accidental trespassers are shot and killed; purposeful trespassers are shot and killed; confused hunters often cross an unfortunate property line during deer season and are shot by armed guards. Because of the frequency of incidents such as this, local police and agricultural commissioners tend to avoid certain wooded segments of the county during deer season. Peace, Love, Dope . . .

These violent incidents occur almost exclusively at commercial farms on unofficial (and wholly illegal—nothing *quasi* about it) gardens set up on timberlands and National Forest property.

"If the Mexican cartels have their hand in anything, it's those farms," Lady Wanda says. "We're an entirely different animal." (I picture a rabbit crossed with a dragon.)

But, as evidenced by the militiaman raid, not even the more peaceable medical marijuana farms like Weckman are immune to violence.

"But these incidents of violence come from the outside. I've never, *ever* had a case of inside violence and neither have most of the medical growers I know," Lady Wanda stresses.

She pauses. She walks among a few of the picnic tables, touching their surfaces. Clearly, she is trapped in 1996, having just finished her last easy cup of coffee.

"It's hard sometimes," she says.

We finish our granola and ready ourselves for the fields. Johanna turns toward the house and sees Robbi the Little Piece of Gristle waving to her from the veranda. On the off-nights when Robbi stays at Weckman, she sleeps in Lady Wanda's house, in a small room on the first floor. She doesn't bear the intense smell of the Pickers. Even Lady Wanda does the yoga. Johanna returns the wave.

"I have to go to work," she says.

I stand with her, hug her, the woman who rode out Chicago with me; who slept in my old room with the drawers full of legless G.I. Joe figures, *Playboy* magazines from the early 1980s, model airplane sets never removed from their plastic; the woman who faced with me my mother's cancer and now a farm subject to raids from air and land. I hug her and want us to be safe, wonder if, somewhere, there is a glossary of terms for the lives we are leading together. Wonder which word would begin it.

"Be careful out there," she says, angling her chin to the fields.

As the rest of the crew finishes and stands, I quickly down the last sip of my cooled coffee. I stare at the empty bottom of my cup, the styrofoam patterned like skin, ringed with grounds, stimulated and worried and sugarless.

Nine

IN THE FIELDS, I begin an unhealthy relationship with the sky—one based on neuroses and the imminent dropping of the other shoe. After the Chicago ordeal, most of my relationships— with sky, with earth, with a plate of food—take this occasional, and maddening, turn.

Every time I hear a mosquito, I expect a helicopter. Every time I hear Bob clicking his tongue a few rows behind me, I expect the cocking of a gun. Forgive me my exaggerations and trespasses, my descents into forehead-wrinkling, hands-in-the-air Woody Allen–ness, and their occasional, and thin, reemergence. Forgive me for not yet finding my own gypsy Melquíades and the poultice that erases bad memories. (Believe me: on Weckman, I tried out numerous "poultices.")

In Chicago, when we felt that the walk to the neighborhood park and swing set was too much, Johanna and I would sit on my parents' front steps biting our lips, at once dreading the next day and looking forward to any further information regarding the third biopsy, the fifth PET scan, the fourteenth unexpected side-effect. The late nights were cool, but not cool enough for my parents to shut their bedroom windows. Johanna and I had to keep our voices low. (I promise: after another weepy Chicago section like this, I will reward you with a song—maybe something by Steppenwolf.)

In a suburb of Chicago, she found a massage therapy job; I found work as an assistant sommelier at an Italian restaurant. Typically, I wouldn't get off work until after midnight, my breath laced with one of the restaurant's homemade flavored grappas—anise, pineapple, five-spice.

We would sit on those front steps, staring into the terrible outside houselights that my parents' across-the-street neighbor would leave on, even during the day; lights that came through my old bedroom window, keeping Johanna and me awake half the night—so bright that even the autographed eight-by-ten glossy of Ryne Sandberg complained, the maimed G.I. Joe figures forgetting their limblessness in the face of the shitty brilliance. At the base of the steps, the maple tree shook in the late-night wind, the branches that I used to climb as a child long since cut down by the district's parks department— they had evidently begun to hang over the sidewalk, impeding the ever-growing number of tricycle-bound and helmeted toddlers, not a single one of them on their way to becoming Dolph Lundgren.

On those steps, we would talk, haphazardly and prematurely, about how we had to turn up our collars against this time, against this cancer (I'm treading thin ice here); about how we had to bury our necks in our proverbial overcoats and keep our heads down against the wind. It was our survival tactic. Through the winter, taking the three dogs for below-zero walks around the block, it was our survival tactic. Repetition, then as now, served as false comfort. Watching the largest of the three dogs bury himself in the snow, tongue lolling, pads freezing, we had to force ourselves to laugh, because we felt it was the right thing to do. It was what people would do.

We would sit on those steps, watching the rare car pass under the streetlights' orange pools, force-feeding each other's neuroses, fleshing out the next shoe, poised to drop, preparing ourselves for anything from penny loafer to Reebok Pump, vinyl stiletto to Air Jordan high-top. But we could handle it—we had our collars turned up, our heads down. Helicopter or relapse, we could handle it.

Instead of looking at each other's faces, Johanna and I would stare into the neighbor's houselights, blinding ourselves even while holding hands. We would listen to the junk opera of sump pumps eructing green water over greener lawns. Between each house was a minor flood, a spongy river over which countless neighborhood feuds began. In this neighborhood, if it wasn't cancer, it was an issue with the lawn.

Johanna came to call the place The Sprinkler Capital of the World.

Some nights, lolling on the concrete steps, Johanna would ask, "Where are we going to go from here?"

While melodramatic, this is no lie.

Other nights, it was my turn to ask.

Then, we would turn our backs on those evil lights and walk heavily into the house. Some nights, we would try to make each other laugh by dropping our pants and mooning the neighborhood. Some nights, it worked.

Opening my parents' front door, we would have to step over Kodiak, the largest of the three dogs, the billowing white, two-hundred-pound Great Pyrenees. We would pet him, kiss him, push our faces as far as we could into the deep fur at his neck. Upstairs, in the kitchen, we would pour our drinks into small cups—vodka with pomegranate juice (the latter recommended to my mom by the oncologist)—and take them to the empty cardboard boxes that became our makeshift nightstands. Undressed, we would crawl into our bed that wasn't our bed, my childhood print of a landing airplane holding to the wall over our heads, Alyssa Milano trapped in awkward youth, that fucking King Kong hologram useless without light. We would sip our drinks and watch network television and not fall asleep.

We would wonder, aloud, if we were irreversibly changed. We would say things, without passion, like, *That was a good commercial.*

I scrutinize the edges of clouds, watching for the artificial light of the helicopter. I scrutinize the chest of my shirt, waiting for it to explode with my blood. Charlie the Mechanic, rightfully, thinks I'm nuts. He is sensible and never indifferent, and his skinny, hairy legs, dropping scarred from his cargo shorts, look as if they're so enjoying the fresh air.

"Ya jus' have t' deal with it, brother. Ev'ry once in a while a carpenter'll put a nail through his hand. Y' know?"

"Yeah," I say, shoving the crate of trimmings onto the flatbed, hoping he's not going to say something about Jesus. "It's just that all of a sudden, everyone's telling these scary stories."

Charlie shrugs in a "What Can We Do about It?" sort of way, a shrug that is the luxury of a man who has doubtlessly experienced untold horrors.

I'm glad Johanna is inside the mansion, with her unarmed bottles of lotion. I'm glad she's not out here, exposed. In one way, Weckman Farm is safer than my parents' front steps; in many others, it's not.

If a vigilante militia decides to invade today, I decide that my best defense would involve the act of biting. (In the fields, engaged in very repetitive, very repetitive, very repetitive physical activity, the mind starts to wander, daydream irrationally, okay?) Given my family's penchant for dealing with tragedy via food, I think making a Chemo Breakfast out of an armed militiaman only makes sense. I'm sure there's a buried, if not universal, syllogism in that somewhere. Maybe California is infecting me. This sounds like something their governor would have said in his former life as Commando-Predator-Hunter-Running Man. I put the words *Chemo Breakfast* into the mouth of Arnold Schwarzenegger and smile while scrutinizing the sky.

Eventually, I finish this row and progress toward the row at the bottom of the hill, trimming where Gloria, in her wheelchair, trimmed before me. Her yellow slippers. The tendons poking like piano strings from her feet. The morning remains helicopterless, as does the early afternoon. No one in camouflage bursts from the bushes; no one pulls any triggers or sets anything on fire. Slowly, the cosmos and I begin to reconcile. The scissors lull me into automatic thoughtlessness, the fan leaves dancing like octopi.

Soon, I hear the approaching sound of an engine, but know right away it's not originating from the sky. The sound is too earthbound, too choked with grass. Somewhere, beyond the rows, the Lawnmower Man patrols the grounds with his snaggle-toothed pet, and albeit irrationally, I feel safe again.

A few rows in front of me, Crazy Jeff shouts, "Takin' it off here, boss. Whoo-hoo-hoo!"

"Take it off!" Lance answers, hidden among the rows.

Over the shuffling of my scissor blades, I hear Ruby mutter something interrogative to Lance.

"*Cool Hand Luke*," Lance explains, his snipping overlapping hers.

The two of them must be trimming in the same row. I smile at this thought; despite my uneasiness today at the threat of violence, I am surprised to discover that I am not yet immune to *cute*. Plus, I adore Lance for resurrecting young Paul Newman (and, I suppose, more accurately, young George Kennedy), if only for an instant.

Decidedly uncute, but lusciously pathetic, is Bob's singing. In his row, higher up the hill, his voice finds the place between words and humming, a desire to be heard, but not by any of us. I can't really make out the song over the riding lawnmower's engine, but I think it may be Steppenwolf's "Magic Carpet Ride."

The engine's buzz begins to fill my ears, then fade away, then fill my ears again. Without turning, I believe the Lawnmower Man must be resuming the informal game of chicken we started on Cutting Day, when I so desired that pair of blue rubber-handled clippers. At the bottom of the crop hill, in the first row of plants, I have again made myself vulnerable to this cybernetic beast. When he pulls forward, I can see the green threads of cut grass dance around my head like electrons, feel the wind of the engine flatten the hair on my legs. Decapitating a bud of Grand Daddy Purple, I kick at the base of my trimming crate and turn to face him.

Today, mercifully, the Lawnmower Man wears blue jeans under his black nightshirt. Had he not, I would most certainly be bearing stunned witness to his ample Portobello. The wind lips the white embroidered hem from his knees; for a second, the cloth rides like a hovercraft before redepositing itself over his denim'd thighs. In this second, the sun catches his belt buckle, large as a silver saucer. I think of aliens and hear Crazy Jeff laughing about something, far up in the rows.

On the buckle, in brief, I make out speckles of turquoise and coral, some nebulous design, some stylized arrows, something vaguely human. Up close, even beneath that billowy nightshirt—as overlarge as Hector's tent—I can see that the Lawnmower Man is skinny, but healthy. His reedy arms poke from the cavernous sleeves like a wizard's. I can see also that he's footed with black cowboy boots.

I imagine his sunken stomach pressed against this giant buckle, his ribs struggling to accommodate its size, his sterling center of gravity. Perhaps this buckle's unnecessary largeness holds him to the lawnmower's chair. The chair, beneath his slight frame, resembles a loveseat, the companion cushion taken up with another, slightly more expansive saucer.

On this rattling dish, I make out what appears to be a hot pastrami sandwich—wisps of steam rising like brined ghosts—and a scoop of cottage cheese on the side.

As always, he wears his white cloth-brimmed hat, tied at its middle with a scarlet sash. At first, I mistook this to be a fishing hat, but here, in the bottommost of the pot rows, I can see that it's more elegant than that, perfect for a dinner at a sidewalk bistro. In Fantasyland. From his neck, a beaded necklace dangles, bearing an obscure golden amulet, tottering just above the buckle of his belt. His beard is wonderful today, massive, white, and holy, as if he purchased it during a vacation in Tibet. This beard is his one attempt to match the physicality of Lady Wanda.

Ivory white, the beard hangs to his sternum, covering the necklace's genesis, and arcs upward into a pyramid of a moustache. His lips, two tiny snakes of skin, protrude from the esplanade of facial hair, demure, delicate, surely housing the mummified remains of the most sacred of child pharaohs.

Cascading from beneath his hat, like ropes anchoring a balloon, are two black tendrils of shoulder-length hair, the last refugees of rebellion against inevitable baldness. The darkness of his hair is shocking in conjunction with his beard; he's not a cyborg at all but a human zebra, if only in the follicles.

He shoves the steering wheel left. The green and gold contraption bucks in protest. The engine whines, but the weeds at the base of the crop hill can't get away. As the lawnmower approaches me, armed only with my clipping scissors, I can see the man squinting against the sun. Indeed, the heavens seem to be conspiring with the Pickers in an effort to blind the ungreetable Lawnmower Man. The day, becoming a hot one, throws its light from the thin windshield of Charlie's tractor, from Crazy Jeff's wristwatch, from the zippers of Bob's windbreaker, from the hairless bright youth of Lance's bare orange chest.

Somewhere, a few rows away, the Shepherd's fancy glasses must be sending their light; Ruby smiles, beaming the sheen of her teeth. From the treetops, Hector sends the light of his sniper's scope; from the kitchen, Alex, Emily, and Antonio cast reflections from their chefs' knives; from the Sofa Room, a dozing Gloria drools the brightest of saliva; from Lady Wanda's basement, Robbi catches the light with her yoga mirror; Johanna captures its warmth with massage oil and sends it, unspoken and spousal, to me in the fields, where I can block it, just by raising an arm, from the eyes of the blinded Lawnmower Man. (I think that's everybody except Waldo, inventorywise. Attendance taken.)

Suddenly able to see, he turns his mount to me, my arms stinking and itching and covered in resin. I am part plant, fuzzy with marijuana, crossbred with Swamp Thing. I keep my revolting arm raised, an extension of the Lawnmower Man's hat brim, the shade he needs to see.

My scissors, uplifted like a torch, must be throwing their light to someone else. I picture Charlie in the fields, zapped by this new reflection, tottering to his side while Crazy Jeff laughs.

Fifteen feet from me, the Lawnmower Man's right cowboy boot finds the brake. He brings his machine to a halt. This green-and-gold-painted brute stands still, this offspring of a love triangle between a Jeep, a Volkswagen Bug, and a beach ball. Its blades spin in place, guillotining the heads of the grasses, churning their botanic viscera into the air.

The Lawnmower Man takes his hands from the steering wheel and smooths his beard with both of them. Despite his slightness, his fingers are thick as cigars. A brown beaded bracelet hangs on his right wrist; on his left, the bone white of his skin.

He cuts the mower's engine but doesn't leave his perch. A fly lands on the brim of his hat and, cocksure, looks the world over. The Lawnmower Man reaches into the deep breast pocket of his nightshirt, a kangaroo born the wrong gender, and with its pouch out of place. From it, he withdraws a peeled carrot. He shakes lint from the vegetable, playing the air with the deftness of a drummer. He takes a big orange bite.

Without the engine noise, the fields at Weckman Farm go startlingly silent. Bob lowers the volume on his singing. I can hear now that it *is* "Magic Carpet Ride"—just the chorus, muttered over and over. *Well, you don't know what we can find . . .*

The Lawnmower Man adjusts the hat on his head. The fly stays put, sensing a tolerant soul. Without lifting a wing, it continues its assessment of the human faction of Weckman Farm.

"Nice day," the Lawnmower Man calls, maybe to me, maybe to Charlie, maybe to the heavens.

He has the voice of a man who has lost a lot of weight—a shaved huskiness, a shed skin. I imagine his vocal cords have stretch marks. For such a skinny man, this voice has too much muscle. This is the voice of a linebacker turned poet, a hit man turned organic gardener. This is a voice that cares for the little things, and has the strength to protect them. On the Lawnmower Man's hat, this fly has nothing to worry about.

Up the hill, Charlie tinkers with the lug nuts in the tractor wheels, his back pressed into the rocky strip of Tractor Alley. Bob's singing approaches a whisper. Crazy Jeff does not laugh. Lance says nothing. Ruby sways. The Lawnmower Man considers the silence around him and takes another bite of the carrot. In his mouth, the sound could be the earth cracking like an egg. The man demands to be answered.

"It is," I manage, not nearly as assured as the fly.

"What's that, brother?" Charlie calls from the tractor.

"It is," I say, "a nice day."

I nod to the lawnmower and its rider.

The Lawnmower Man frowns, but in that smiling sort of way. He shifts his hips. He looks as if he'd be more comfortable on a horse.

"Better keep ridin', Lawnmower Man," Charlie jokes, grunting, wrestling with a lug nut. "Stoppin' in the open like that, a helicopter'll get ya."

I wish he didn't say that. The Lawnmower Man raises his carrot to the side of his mouth like a flute. I imagine Charlie behind his trumpet. The fly, hungry, angelic, steps to the edge of his hat brim, appraising this strange orange root.

"I always tell you, Charlie," the Lawnmower Man says, his voice flexing its quadriceps, readying itself for a run, "in security is the likeliest death."

Here, the Lawnmower Man lets loose with the laughter of self-amusement—not a Crazy Jeff *whoo-hoo* kind of laughter, but one that sounds like a lamb calling for its mother.

"Mm-aaa-aaa-aaa, mm-aaa-aaa-aaa . . ."

"Shiiiit," Lance intones from his row.

Again, Ruby mutters something interrogative.

"Just Norman," Lance says to her.

Norman? Could this be the Lawnmower Man's real name? I feel as if I have overheard a secret, delicious and dire. I am attacked with visions of the Dalai Lama and Hitchcock's *Psycho*, and the lamb in his laugh finding that its mother has been renamed *mutton*.

"Eat it, Lance," the Lawnmower Man says, "and give your girl a kiss."

Whether Lance kisses Ruby on command, I do not see. But I hear Charlie laugh, and Crazy Jeff laugh, and see the Lawnmower Man (Norman?) point to all of us with his carrot before finishing it in four sharp bites. He restarts the engine, waves to us with his thick hand, and throws the machine into gear, a tease.

I return the wave and pull the shirt collar from my neck. Sweat runs over my chest, forcing a chill when the wind blows. The Lawnmower Man turns his chariot for Lady Wanda's mansion, his tiny winged sidekick enjoying the free ride, magic carpet or not.

139

Ten

IN 2005 MENDOCINO COUNTY'S economic profits
garnered by all legal endeavors amounted to about 2.5 billion dollars.
Approximately 70 million dollars of this total came from the timber
industry, 62 million dollars from the wine industry. Comparatively,
the economic profits garnered by the marijuana industry amounted
to about 1.7 billion dollars.

"And that doesn't account for the profits made off us by the local
businesses, dude," Norman tells Johanna and me.

Yes, the Lawnmower Man's name is Norman. Yes (not that it was
obvious), he is Lady Wanda's live-in boyfriend. I imagine the sex,
search for the adjectives, come up short, and decide to spare you. A
few key nouns, though: beard, rhinestones, theater curtains of arm
fat, tenderness. Johanna said it best in a phrase native to her home
country, loosely translated as . . . *like a bulldog facedown in a bowl
of corn porridge*.

Norman also serves as one of the heretofore faceless messengers
who drive into the nearby (again, not so near) towns to purchase
the personalized supplies for the harvesting crew. In his eyes alone
is a gloomy peace that could only have come from endurance and a
nomadic lifestyle—surely, Norman survived scurvy on the beaches
of Cape Verde, cholera in Delhi, encephalitis in Ikuno. His eyes
bear the weight of dead leaves, leaking the secrets of some kind of
afterlife, a spirit world that he belongs to more than this one—he

seems to be waiting out the life of the body, having moved beyond it, but he's well-stocked with patience.

Johanna and I are riding with him, only slightly less patient, in a red Jeep Wrangler with a rusted chassis into which he has installed a front bench seat from a defunct Chevrolet Celebrity. This must be the closest roadworthy vehicle to his beloved riding lawnmower. I am plastered against the passenger door by the bodies of two lovely people. Space is tight, but nice. Johanna takes the middle. We've been told that, at some point during the harvest ("Always after Cutting Day," Lady Wanda stressed), Norman gets his kicks out of trucking newbies into one of the local small towns "to witness the transformation," as he says.

"No one really knows how much the harvest season boosts the local economy," Norman explains to us, the Jeep vibrating over the narrow dirt road leading out of Weckman Farm.

It feels surprisingly good to burst these confines, akin to disembarking an airplane after a redeye to Venus. The air seems different, more prodigious, yellower.

Norman, for the second day in a row, wears his long black nightshirt (unwashed) with blue jeans (a new pair) and black cowboy boots (his only pair). The same belt buckle marks his waist. Now, sitting only one body-length away from him, I can see that it bears a bejeweled version of the Native American "End of the Trail" design—an exhausted Native warrior sitting hunched on an exhausted horse. Here, on his belt, Norman somehow fuses himself with both my mother and a pockmarked American history.

Not as pockmarked, but certainly blemished, is this road. Johanna and I have not been along this road since we first came to work on the farm. After driving for over a mile, Norman wrestles with the converted Jeep's steering wheel, his elbows raised. He smells like cumin. I can't imagine what I smell like.

We approach the first of four locked gates that deter entrance to Lady Wanda's way-way-way-off-the-beaten-path property. Quickly braking, Norman hops from the car and twists the combination lock securing the iron gate, his hair tendrils lifting into the wind. Flakes of barely blue paint fall from the metal to the earth as he pushes the gate open with a splitting creak. He jumps back into the Jeep, drives us beyond, parks again, and relocks the gate behind him. We will repeat this process for the next two gates.

At the final gate, we approach a command station, not unlike those posted at the entrances to state parks. The man inside, armed to be sure, recognizes the Jeep and waves to Norman. Norman does not return the wave.

"Randy," he says in quiet acknowledgement.

Randy, a thirtysomething man with a handlebar moustache stiff enough to do chin-ups on, steps from the booth and unlocks the final gate for us. This is the first time both Johanna and I have seen this man, his post about three miles along a barely travelable road from our darling Residents' Camp. I wonder briefly about his life, the wine he would keep on his bed stand and sip, deep into the night, as his wife, twenty years his senior, snores like an antelope next to him, dreaming of Bora Bora. I'm guessing a bottle of Nebbiolo.

And that's about it for Randy. He's seasoning. An ingredient that adds a small bit of flavor but disappears into the fabric of the whole dish.

After passing through this final gate, we drive for another mile, until we reach a small paved road, upon which we see no other cars.

"I forgot how out of the way we are," I say to Norman, or, if I didn't really say it, I thought it; or, if I didn't really think it, *aaayyy, what's the big deal?* Anyhow, as usual, Johanna said it better.

"I'm surprised we don't have to have a DNA test or something to reenter."

Norman laughs, "Yes. How would we go about that, dude? We'd have to be like these scientists. These arrogant fuckers, you know? They called junk DNA *junk* because they didn't know what function it served. It was later discovered that junk DNA is *everything*."

These Normanisms are, for the most part, accurately rendered, as I got into the habit of keeping a pen and folded-up loose-leaf paper in my pocket, trying to be discreet.

Johanna and I nod. We have discovered that Norman, when not atop his lawnmower, has quite a bit to say.

"But, of course, as you know, they want to wash my mouth out with soap," Norman continues.

We approach a stop sign, take a right, and snake along a road just as narrow, just as carless.

"Sometimes," Norman says, "when we bring people up here for the first time, we have them wear blindfolds."

"Really?" I ask.

"Yeah, dude. We have to," he says, pauses, and then continues. "When my grandmother washed my mouth out with Ivory soap, I felt like I had been introduced to whale blubber pie."

"Hm," Johanna responds.

"That's a joke, dude," he says. "Mm-haaa-aaa."

Like the Jeep, like his lawnmower, Norman leaps among fragments and associations, pressing his own gas pedal, feeding his velocity in narrative. I stare out the window.

He proceeds to tell us about how the harvest unofficially affects the local economy, one hand descending from the steering wheel to his belt buckle, as if the etched warrior breathes the words into his palm.

"It's all unofficial, dude. There's not much official, anymore. Never really was, I guess."

Every year, during harvest season, Norman tells us, the populations of the local towns swell, incorporating ten to fifty times the normal amount of people. Many of these people come to work on the farms; many come for the resulting social scene. Local businesses begin stocking marijuana paraphernalia; other businesses—restaurants and retail shops—open their doors only during the annual harvest, further supporting the nomadic lifestyle of the service and kitchen staff.

"They've got to support these scenes," Norman says as we come upon the first stoplight of our journey. A relic from another age. Still, on both sides of the road, we are flanked by redwoods, the asphalt shrouded in shade, the sun buried behind their skyscraping trunks.

Norman tells us that the smell of the marijuana farms—the smell of marijuana itself—permeates these towns during the season.

"There's a wave of tolerance," Norman says, "but there's still full-on harassment from the cops. They're on the prowl. You can *not* fuck up when you drive. You can't be missing any *screws* from your fucking license plate."

Norman tells us that many people deodorize their clothes and car before going into town (though we did not). If we were driving with any marijuana (we are not), Norman would have to be carrying a certificate detailing how much Weckman Farm is allowed to transport at a given time.

"Every time I make a delivery to the dispensaries, I better make sure I have it on me," he says. "But not today. We don't smell too bad, and we're not traveling with any, so we should be fine. It's quite something. For a handful of months, it's quite something. Don't worry too much about it. It's a very friendly scene."

It *is* quite something. Notable musicians travel from larger California cities and other states to play the local bars and coffeehouses; artists dapple the streets, selling their pottery, weavings, paintings, jewelry; poets stand on crates and read their work beneath the streetlights; jugglers pass their hats.

"Last year, there was this guy lying on a bed of nails," Norman tells us. "Jeremiah, his name was. He put a coffee can out for donations and made enough cash to take the rest of the year off. I haven't seen him this year, though."

I look to Johanna. People in Chicago just don't do this: make their living—a very good living—lying on nails.

Precisely how much the marijuana harvest affects the local economy remains undetermined. Growers rarely deposit their profits into local banks, especially since the federal government requires the bank to file deposit reports for amounts exceeding ten thousand dollars. Further, there's no way to tally exactly how much of the marijuana economy's 1.7 billion dollars in profits is redeposited back into Mendocino County's legal business economy.

But, turning right at the light onto a road speckled with a few other cars now, which also seem relics of an earlier age—nay—a far more hectic future, Norman tells us that he knows of many legitimate local businesses whose survival depend on the pot harvest.

"Without it, and the buzz, and the scenesters, we'd be surrounded by ghost towns," he says. "The economists know it, the people here know it, but the government, dude . . . But the government can change. Look at Barry Goldwater. You really gotta admire a man for going crazy with plaque in his blood. Especially if he avoids World War Three. Mm-haaa-aaa-aaa."

I want to say something intelligent here, prove myself to Norman, whose obscure knowledge and barrage of references delight me (not that Goldwater is so obscure). Maybe I can regurgitate something from the National Geographic Channel, or Animal Planet. Something about the reproductive system of the prairie dog, or velocity and how it applies to wormholes.

For all of the pro-marijuana socialites that descend upon these otherwise sleepy towns, there is a contingency of anti-marijuana protesters who travel here as well. They preach their gospel from their own crates.

"There's always one dude who shouts in the streets about how he kicked drugs, and everybody else should follow suit because he's *been there*," Norman says.

I nod and breathe in the air through the open windows. Johanna shifts her weight between Norman and me. The air here, miles outside of Weckman, is decidedly less vegetal, full of concrete and a bit of industry. But it smells good. On leaving the farm for the first time in weeks, I realize how claustrophobic the same air can be, even if that air is cleaner than most. Johanna puts one hand on my leg and another on Norman's. I can tell she's finally found her western United States father figure.

He continues, "If you stopped taking drugs because this lying bastard stopped taking drugs, that's not a good thing. That's shaky at best."

I laugh, but Norman does not, and because of this, arrest my laugh midway. Johanna drums on our legs.

Norman strokes his beard and looks at Johanna, smiling.

"But what the fuck do I know?" he says. "Ask anybody in town, dude. I'm the original brat. This self-indulgent brat . . . in addition to being the Gothic Santa Claus of Loneliness."

I ready myself to laugh again but can't go through with it.

Johanna touches the end of his beard, and I take a deep breath of this fresh, dirtier air and smile.

Norman says, "Mm-haaa-aaa," bemused by himself.

The redwoods thin to shorter, skinnier trees; a few vineyards poke from the distance. I begin to hear, through the open Jeep window, the jangle of an amplified electric guitar. After the acoustic instruments of Weckman Farm, it's nice to hear something that requires plugging in.

I'M WONDERING HERE if I'm giving Norman far too much attention, too much page space. Doesn't Charlie the Mechanic or Lance or Crazy Jeff—hell, even Gloria, Hector, the German Shepherd, Ruby, or Lady Wanda herself—deserve this kind of attention, presented like a series of entries in some bizarro *Bartlett's Quotations*? Is there an (albeit intriguing) irrelevancy in detailing at such length our journey into town with him? I'm hoping this strange irrelevancy adds spice, and thus makes these scenes relevant.

With Norman, in town, Johanna and I were asked to cope with a scene both beautiful in its freewheeling openness and maddening in its commitment to weirdness and lack of engagement with anything as real (and as human) as cancer. Can fighting for one's life be an art? Can fleeing from such a fight be art criticism? Or is that just another maddening commitment to weirdness?

I touch Johanna's leg as Norman perfectly parallel-parks the Jeep between two white Volkswagen Buses. She turns to me with the eyes of a woman who has no idea how, or why, coming from a small town in northern Sweden, she now finds her ass planted between the great, humanized Lawnmower Man and a husband who drags her from joy, to tragedy, to weirdness in rarefied Northern California. This is surely a tour of American life to render the Swedish-language brochures limp. On her leg, warming beneath khaki capris, my hand evolves from touch to tickle.

"Mm-haa-haa," Johanna mimics, and Norman's laugh sounds so good (and a little sexy) in her mouth.

I want to kiss her hard, press her up against Norman as if he were a paper-thin wall, undress her and kiss her, make the noise of the metronome. Norman nods as if he knows what I'm thinking, and I wouldn't be surprised if he did. At a certain age, in certain people, wisdom confuses itself with clairvoyance.

I want to laugh too, and I want him to laugh. When sealed into a confined farm space for a number of weeks, there is a giddiness to leaving, to going anywhere, exciting or mundane—the bank, the post office, the library—a giddiness illogical and irrepressible.

Irrepressible also, is this town. It houses a wild cultural experiment driven not *by* marijuana but because of marijuana. I try to picture it during the off season, reclaimed by the locals—a placid town that smells of industry and salt, a few people walking their dogs, just them and the weather. Now, though, the streets are lined with scenesters, pot harvest folk emptying their dramatic reserves—faces made up mime-white, devil-red. People walking on their feet and hands, stilts and pogo sticks; contortionists threatening to kiss their own asses; breasts contained and exposed, sometimes hidden with Rapunzel-length hair, sometimes with blue body paint; fantasy and reality leashed to the same tether.

A person (man or woman, I can't tell) plays the saxophone badly while dressed in an alien costume—glittery silver jumpsuit, full green face-mask with a slot just wide enough to accommodate the instrument's mouthpiece. Oddly gloved, the Martian hands dance over the keys, mother-of-pearl meeting rubber suction cup. The alien has upturned a black Area 51 ball cap on the pavement at its green feet. Already, just after lunchtime, it is overflowing with dollar bills.

The Jeep's window acts as a movie screen, releasing, in pumps of human film over a flickering bulb of sunlight, ribbons of celluloid that Fellini would have killed to have captured.

Music from one bar merges with the music of another, this chaotic symbiosis providing the soundtrack for the marvelous supersonics of the sidewalk. People fuse with reptile and flower, acrylic and yarn: latex masks, leis of roses, war paint, peace paint, homemade wigs. I am bearing witness to the genesis of a new generation of nursery rhymes; like the old ones, they just barely conceal their adulthood below a surface of dizzy youth, fueled by something desperate but nevertheless full of life.

"This is awesome," Johanna says.

I nod, unsure if this is the good kind of awe or the bad kind. For example, I am in awe of Jeffrey Dahmer's killing practices. Norman spins the car key inward, kills the Jeep's engine. This fat-handed skinny man struggles to hold onto his key chain.

Just outside the window, a tall, knobby man in a loincloth lies on his back, on top of a yellow Slip 'n Slide, the lawn-bound backyard waterslide that was the envy of every kid in suburban Chicago. It was on a Slip 'n Slide that I, breaking into puberty, saw my first breast as a sexual thing. Amy Crossin. She was three years older than any of us (always will be), spilling out of a baggy red bikini top after a reckless headfirst dive. This event remained famous among the neighborhood boys, long after Amy moved to Oregon to live with her grandparents.

This lanky man disturbs my long-dormant memory of her, makes it embarrassing and, somehow, Roman. A small sprinkler rakes fingernails of water over his body, hairless, glistening. I do not mention Amy to Johanna, if only because I'm afraid of what Norman will say—doubtless, something about a historical penis, and its iconic psychopomp.

Instead, I ask her, "Do you think that's Robbi's boyfriend?"

In this question, Norman takes no interest. Johanna elbows me in the ribs as we step from the car. The lanky man bites at the air—a greyhound going after the horseflies. I wonder who his family is, and what conversations he has with them when visiting for Thanksgiving.

The sprinkler's hose snakes around the back of a head shop, with or without the cooperation of the managers. For sale, in the display window, are pot bongs of blown glass, pipes the length of a leg, pipes the length of a thumb, books on growing marijuana indoors and hydroponically, psychedelic bumper stickers, wallets made of hemp, sewn with decals both Asian and Jamaican. This is a full global assault of yin, yang, and Bob Marley, and I'm not sure how long I can take it. I can listen to the jangling of hair-bangles and skirt-bells for just so long before lunacy sets in.

To the left of the shop's doors, a man in a starched white shirt and black pants stands, literally, on a soapbox. (Well, to be honest, a Clorox Bleach box.) He harangues an ambivalent crowd. Straight out of a 1930s government-funded cautionary tale, the man spews demonic evidence pointing to marijuana's designation as the Devil's Weed. His sweat stains rival those of Pickers on Cutting Day, though his rasp has nothing on Charlie the Mechanic's, his mania, nothing on Crazy Jeff's.

"Rightful!" he shouts, his big glasses falling from the bridge of his nose.

He readjusts them on his face, not with his hands, which are clutching beanless (and therefore soundless) maracas, but with an upward fling of his neck. His blonde hair is slicked back and his face is red.

"Hateful!" he continues. "Don't let them make *yooouuuu* this way!"

He catches my eye, and I look away.

On the other side of the shop doors, standing behind the Slip 'n Slide Man's gunboat feet, is a small woman in a blue bikini top and aerated ankle-length skirt, also blue. She is long-toed and barefoot, her nails painted an end-of-the-rainbow gold. She juggles dice, the three tiny cubes spinning in the air—a drunken daredevil game of craps. Beautifully, these two ignore the Maraca Man. Though they don't look at each other, there is something familial between them. Maybe they're husband and wife, brother and sister.

"Mmm-haa-aaa," Norman mutters, sliding his body from Jeep to street. "Willie and Rain. They're here every year."

He gestures to the Slip 'n Slide Man and his die-juggling companion. They don't seem to notice him, lost in what I guess has to be called their performance.

"So," I begin, "what's their act?"

"Only flames!" the Maraca Man scolds from the other side of the doorway as the sprinkler continues to pump its water.

"Dude," Norman answers me. "They're calling upon the athletes of Ethiopia."

Johanna turns to him. My cerebrum mouths *What the fuck?* to my medulla oblongata, which responds by increasing my blood pressure, shortening my breath. Is this merely senseless chaos?

"Ethiopia?" she asks.

"Same thing every year," he says. "They correspond with these sibling runners over there . . . by mail, I guess. I forget his name, but the brother is this Ethiopian long-distance runner who trains by lying in a dugout near some river and back-floating. One time, he fell asleep and woke up thirty-five miles later. His sister runs the one-hundred-meter dash and meditates before each event by juggling dice."

Again, Norman gestures to them, actually waves, but again, his greeting remains unrequited.

The Maraca Man shouts, "And we all know that this is the only place that smoke can take us!"

With a silent maraca, he mimics a plane going down, crashing at his wing-tipped feet.

I bite at my fingernails, dazed, sun-washed. A bedsheet of pot smoke hovers above us, perhaps the ingredient required to make sense of the chaos. Despite Norman's warnings of an overzealous police presence, every squad car we see merely slows down, watches the street scene for a few seconds, and moves on. I suppose during harvest season, amid this atmosphere, tolerance is forced upon them. Smoke and nudity are, even to the law, gentler than blood. At least in California. As one cop car passes, two young men in assless pants race after it. Their smooth cheeks bob like a spirit orb in quadruplicate.

Johanna clings to my side, then pulls away, torn between the comfort of the old and the electricity of the new. Norman wanders unaffected, his senses accustomed to the assault. His arms slither at his sides, as if craving a larger belly to fold themselves over—perhaps the one Norman himself used to have.

He guides us along the sidewalk. We pass a girl in a back brace giving henna tattoos for five bucks. She has a gorgeous porcelain face, but her posture is ruined. When she concentrates on her work, she looks as if she needs to have a good cry but hasn't yet had the time to let it out. I realize now: Who the fuck am I to say these people have no engagement with real and human tragedy? Who am I—some asshole who with his wife fled from his mother's sickbed to a fucking *marijuana farm*—to say what is and what isn't a valid response to misfortune?

Behind us, barely audible now, the Maraca Man shouts, "Garters!"

We stop in front of an old man doing caricatures of passersby as hallucinogenic fish. Every so often, he puts down his pens and sips from Alka-Seltzer-and-lime-spiked water. I can only imagine the homemade birthday cards he sends to his estranged grandchildren. Norman points to his easel.

"One year, I was a hammerhead shark," he tells us. "I never sat for the fucker again. Mmm-haaa-aaa."

We walk. A sandaled boy sits unchaperoned behind a dirt box, selling pubic sprouts of Red Russian kale. As much as the crippled henna tattoo girl needed to cry, this boy needs to laugh. He watches, with bored eyes, the crowd pass him by. His cardboard sign advertises, in decidedly adult handwriting, five cents a sprout.

"Hello," Johanna says to him.

His smile is amazing.

A few yards further up the sidewalk, a trio of twentysomethings (two women and a man), clad only in elaborate body paint, sell entry ("Over 18 only!") to their naked haunted house. This is a small tent cloaked in opaque black cloth, a miniature and far more titillating version of Lady Wanda's food tent. The two women are painted as matching birds of prey. The man, swathed in pale red, can only be their worm. The archetypal early bird implications are too tempting to resist but too obvious to say aloud.

To Johanna, I speculate instead about spider-themed hand puppets leaping from the haunted dark and stirring, in one way or another, the patrons into ecstatic submission. Dramatically, she licks her lips.

"Sounds like it's worth the six bucks," she says.

Norman walks two strides ahead of us, the wind lifting the night-shirt from his body, as if a naked haunted tent all its own. He is a sorcerer walking on air, our unofficial tour guide to the world just outside Weckman. Behind him, we progress, if you can call it that.

We pass an old woman who, for three-fifty, will diagnose your madness. She sits alone at her foldout bridge table, reading an old issue of *Better Homes and Gardens*. Next to her, two girls in string bikinis offer to rub suntan lotion on our backs for eight bucks apiece (discounted from ten, their sign assures us). Their skin, still so elastic, has the appearance of a dolphin's—at once nauseatingly attractive and unattractive.

Johanna grumbles something about how they give massage therapy a bad name. Norman, looking over his shoulder (at us or them, I can't tell), laughs.

We come to a shop front, its entrance hidden behind a curtain of beads. The chalkboard sign outside advertises "Mirror Art." Norman explains that this involves stepping into a dressing room of sorts, disrob-ing, and squatting over a floor mirror. Patrons are invited to examine, dwell on, and meditate over "the secrets of their undersides." Then they dress and, from memory, publicly sculpt their hidden places in clay, which Belinda, the shop owner, will then fire in a kiln and cool. Patrons paint their baked "pieces" in a variety of colors. Belinda is most certainly not the dominatrix I imagine her to be, but I lack the courage to step beyond the beads and find out. Johanna, joyful, shakes her head.

"You ever go into that one, Norman?" she asks.

"Oh, god, no," he laughs, running his sturdy hands over his torso. "I've lost my magic. But I don't want my fucking dukedom back. That would be trouble."

"I think it's trouble already," I smile.

The wind shifts the beaded doorway. I squint, trying to see inside, but to no avail. The hidden stays hidden.

"Mmm-haa-aaa. Wanda did it once years ago. The Twat Squat,

she calls it. Mmm-haa-aaa. The result was this wreath she put up at Christmas. This wreath as a nest—takes the idea of mother and puts a dead zero in its center. Mmm-haa-aaa."

"Since when is an opening a zero?" Johanna challenges.

Norman laughs again, and blushes. He starts talking about "the days of Prospero and Miranda . . ." and a *Nova* TV special he saw about Joan of Arc.

We continue, slowly, along the sidewalk, the music scribbling its blues, folk, rockabilly, funk. The aural melting pot is surprisingly listenable, a confirmation of the multiplication table and the success of exponents, at least when pumped through speakers.

We pass a white man in a turban charming a plastic snake from a pink basket. He wears a gold wedding band on his left ring finger. Beyond him, a long-haired, shirtless bodybuilder wears a necklace of chicken bone. He poses, his hands on his hips, his palms facing downward, in a textbook front-lat spread. The "Hello My Name Is . . ." tag on his left pectoral reads "Konan the Fucked-Up Barbarian." (Yes, he spells Conan with a *K*.) Johanna points to him.

To Norman and me she whispers, "Small dick."

Norman and I laugh like two bleating sheep.

A man dressed as Neptune (the planet, not the god) invites passersby to "be the distant sun," revolving lazily around him for fifty cents.

"I'm not revolving around a gas giant," Norman says.

A small girl in a white dress and garland of white flowers (she must be Neptune's daughter) takes a Polaroid and hands it to the patron upon completing "the revolution." Johanna speculates that the girl must be home-schooled.

We walk on, motion the only thing that keeps us from the underworld. A woman dressed as a heavily mascaraed corpse plays a toy harp. A dwarf in a bowler hat stands on a bar stool, extending a long metal pole into the air. For a dollar, you can stand beneath his reach and, for sixty seconds, protect yourself from imminent lightning. (There's not a cloud in the sky.) An a cappella barbershop quintet dressed like the Marx Brothers strains to be heard over the live music of the bars and coffeehouses. They do an impeccable version of "You Are So Beautiful." Chico, the baritone, is the best singer (or maybe just the loudest) of the bunch. As always, Gummo and Zeppo take the back seat. Johanna and I hold hands.

Together, we sing along, "tooo meeee!"

The quintet smiles. Groucho has a cardboard sign strung around his neck, imploring, in black magic marker, "Where's Cousin Karl?" Harpo advertises ten-cent haircuts with a pair of giant plastic scissors.

As we come to The Verse, Norman's oasis of choice and caffeine, we pass a staid man in his seventies, wearing a pinstriped apron and straw hat, selling hot dogs. Simply selling hot dogs. His red and yellow awning reads, "Snacks above Reproach."

AFTER WORKING AS a bus driver and as an engineer for Boeing, Norman, as a slightly younger man, worked the streets of this town, faking antiques. Though this was only about ten years ago, I can't help but cast Norman, and this town, in sepia. Surely, the local law enforcement, all carrying six-guns, waxed moustaches, and an Earpian air, constantly threatened his sidewalk busker operation. Surely, only ten years ago, this town was a town of tumbleweeds. Marijuana had not yet eclipsed the Old West vices of moonshine and opium.

We sit at a table in what I imagine to be an ex-brothel—one in which the ladies bore beehive hairdos and red dresses pluming with expensive fabric. We are in The Verse coffeehouse, hugging an open window. The place is drenched in gilded treble clefs and enough wood paneling to make the redwoods cringe. The afternoon house band is mercifully electric—four local celebrities who play, according to our benightshirted host, "the best surf gospel this side of Copenhagen, dude."

I imagine the treble clefs detaching themselves from the wallpaper, unraveling like carpets. A few hours with Norman and my rare sober mind has already adopted some of his erratics. But this is a man whose personality and wardrobe are so firmly placed outside of our Chicago experience that I can't help but thank my lucky stars that

I can, at least for a little while, sit at the edge of his beard. In fact, it is only his beard that returns me to Chicago by association. It is the facial-bound version of Kodiak the Great Pyrenees.

Norman drums his fingers against the table. I remember this: he was a serious table-drummer. A mess of tarot cards lies pressed beneath the clear glass tabletop, the wrought iron legs holding the piece of furniture in place, and our three coffee cups upon it. This is not the dishwater coffee of the Granny Annie's variety that sustained us in its delightful classic diner weakness through many a Chemo Breakfast. This, like Durban Poison, as Lance might say, is some concentrated shit.

In harvest seasons past, The Verse, along with many independent businesses in Northern California, had converted itself into an Amsterdam-style marijuana (and coffee) bar. To barely skirt the law (miniskirt the law?), such seasonal businesses took a page from the private clubs, providing membership cards to medical marijuana patients only. These patients would sign an affidavit naming the club as their lawful caregiver, allowing a place like The Verse to distribute marijuana to, and sometimes for, them. These clubs would routinely possess anywhere from sixteen to six thousand members.

Many of the Northern California pot clubs had security guards, and specific rules about smoking, or not smoking, on the property. Many clubs offered their patrons leather-bound menus detailing the available strains of marijuana as if beers on tap. Additionally, these menus routinely offered various strains of hash and hash oils, marijuana-infused breads, teas, ice creams, candies, and pastries.

"It was great," Norman tells us, slurping his latte. "The marijuana industry was finally beginning to self-regulate. Local businesses doubled as dispensaries during the harvest season. And now, it's pretty much a mass moratorium. But who knows how long it will last . . . this time."

During the current moratorium on such dispensaries, both seasonal and year-round, the Americans for Safe Access (ASA) marijuana advocacy group is attempting to establish specific regulations for these patients' clubs in an effort to spawn a mass and grand reopening. One can only imagine: *Buy one joint, get one joint of equal or lesser value free!* Because in this industry, like any other, a few bad apples spoil things for the whole bunch, the ASA hopes to enumerate a doctrine that will appeal to the local governments. This doctrine will include ways to register and identify patients, and the prescribing doctors, and will attempt to suffuse the industry with a measure of uniformity.

Many pro-dispensary locals champion this effort, while others dismiss it as unnecessary playing of the government's game. The latter faction argues that devoting energy to detailed bureaucratic regulation is an example of skewed priorities; that there's no way that the ASA's doctrine could ever be uniformly enforced; that it's the same historical beating of the same historical drum.

Many believe that the true success story of legal marijuana dispensing (if there is to be one) lies in the hands of the doctors. If doctors were to prescribe marijuana judiciously, and in written form, many believe that amiable regulation is possible. Others pessimistically (they might say, realistically) counter that there will always be some official to challenge the previously established notions of *judicious* and *amiable*.

Law enforcement has prosecuted doctors for prescribing marijuana indiscriminately, while these doctors defend the prudence of their actions. Law enforcement will sometimes send an undercover agent to investigate these small-town dispensaries. In cases, the owners have been arrested, threatened with life imprisonment, their shops, like Weckman Farm, raided and shut down. Many times, these owners are acquitted, their shops reopened, their bank accounts tens of thousands of dollars lighter. Where does all that money go?

Many doctors complain that these undercover agents judge the health of a dispensary patient via mere visual assessment. Fearing prosecution, a number of California doctors have stopped prescribing marijuana to patients who they believe are in need. In the "few bad apples" vein, some doctors have been known to cater to a marijuana-loving clientele, signing medical slips for money. The more conservative of the prescribing doctors, along with the ASA, hope that specific regulation can help the local law enforcement distinguish between the bad and good apples. The Pink Ladies and the Red Deliciouses, the Spartans and the Snows, the McIntoshes and the Honeycrisps.

Even those who believe ASA's efforts may be in vain also tend to believe that some form of regulation will, eventually, be necessary, perhaps if, and/or when, federal law comes around. But mass cooperation is always a slippery, and elusive, slope. A Slip 'n Slide on a mountainside, if you will.

For many, the question remains: How can we legislate ethics?

"What will steal maturity from us," Norman says, "is the government. And art! Still, the Measure P babies have a point."

In November of 2006, many miles south of Weckman Farm, the citizens of Santa Barbara voted to pass a bill called Measure P. In effect, this measure declared that marijuana use for persons over age eighteen, whether medical or recreational, was to be given minimal priority by local law enforcement.

Despite the bill, many locals (dispensary owners among them) claim that the George W. Bush administration had been federally cracking down on marijuana use, putting pressure on local governments and law enforcement agencies. As the Obama administration has had its hands full, it has been difficult to find the time necessary to revise such strong-arm tactics in the smaller towns. As such, status bestowed upon such clubs is increasingly becoming a criminal one, in spite of the pro–medical marijuana propositions that thirteen states have passed as of 2009 (many of which are maddeningly vague when it comes to regulation in practice). Small-town police have been giving increased attention to these Amsterdam-style deviances, however arguably benign. There are those who argue that allowing the dispensaries and farms to operate as "legal" businesses—keeping records, paying taxes—will cause the availability of unregulated rogue marijuana to decrease at street level; that this is something that should make the police happy.

At any rate, in recent years, The Verse has remained just a coffee shop, one in which the occasional patron will light up a joint, tolerated or unnoticed.

"Dude," Norman says. "The state laws are in conflict with the federal laws. There is no mass understanding of marijuana law. When we're breaking it, we're not. When we're not, we are. But sometimes, people get scared. Now we all have to mourn the eccentric old shrimp fisherman who didn't have a soul, but a dog."

Johanna and I glance at each other, then turn away, fearing inappropriate laughter. With Norman, one's not sure if it's safe to laugh until he does. Either that, or if he injects the post-pause caveat, *That's a joke, dude.*

Behind Norman, the clinking of mugs and breath of the cappuccino steamer are drowned out by the sounds of a greaser guitarist with Carl Perkins eyebrows, tuning his instrument through an amplifier.

"But even now, really, if a place wanted to do it, they could, *legally.* As long as they had a fucking business license," Norman continues, raising his voice over the plucking of the G string.

He tells us: even these "legal" businesses have a history of being shut down via prosecution, only to reopen some months later, only to be shut down again.

"The paperwork is on our side and the paperwork is against us," Norman says, referencing the various licenses needed to grow and sell medical marijuana either to, or from, a dispensary.

As a result, nobody really knows—not the police, not Lady Wanda, not the owners of The Verse—what they're permitted to be doing. Regulations seem to be defined only by individual arrests and court dates. And chances are, a week later, another arrest and court date will contradict the regulations laid out in the one prior.

"Ask Wanda," Norman says. "It's all like a big fake fight. It can be a real labor. But there's desire in labor. There's desire for the end of desire."

I wait for a Taoist quote, filtered through the udders of a birthing cow—in short, a typical Normanism—but he simply, for a moment, stares at the backs of his hands.

Norman's fingers escalate their table-tapping. The Verse's house band comes to life behind him, forcing the outside street scene to the background. The patrons sip their caffeinated drinks around us. For the moment, The Verse is joint-less.

The guitarist, now in tune, picks a surf melody, deep-frying what is basically medicine-show gospel. He sniffs the air as if missing something. At the microphone, a tall man and tall woman exchange a God-fearing call-and-response, he adorned with a yellow mohawk, she sporting a shaved head. They stick out their tongues, stopping just short of a pornographic kiss. In their mouths, I expect to see piercings, something metallic, but see only soft pink muscle unadorned, teeth so square and white The Verse must offer them a dental plan, or they discovered that rare Clorox toothpaste before it was yanked from the shelves for tasting like sodium hypochlorite. The lead guitarist hides behind Coke-bottle sunglasses and a blue crushed-velvet jumpsuit, a human threesome between Elvis Presley, Billy Graham, and Evel Knievel.

Johanna bobs her head. Norman stops his finger-drumming. Apparently, he wanted to predict the music, not engage it. Despite limiting themselves to the sale of coffee (still legal, for now), The Verse and its house band drip with covert exclusivity. Somehow admitted, I bob my head too. The silent sign of the cult.

The rear of the stained wood stage is occupied by an obese bassist in a cardboard Burger King crown, a dusty drummer, and dustier keyboardist. All three grit their teeth, affecting underbites. Occasionally, the spastic keyboardist leaps from his stool and plays the higher keys with the heel of his silver spray-painted combat boot. His pinky fingernails must be three inches long.

Though we sit near an open window, and the wind and light from the street penetrate the place, The Verse has a decidedly insular feel. Increasingly, I am surprised we didn't have to utter a password or demonstrate a handshake to get in. Bookshelves lined with broken-spined paperbacks hug the yellowing walls, Joseph Heller sharing space with Danielle Steel. I envision a book cover: Fabio and Joan Collins riding a missile bareback into 1940s Germany.

Candlelit torch-style lanterns protrude from The Verse's walls. Iron, black, and gothic, the lamps recall human hands forever trapped in painted plaster. The ghosts of The Verse's bygone dispensary days?

The bar itself is like the tables, the remnants of an ancient poker game on the Day of the Dead. Though merely wood and lacquer, the bar seems in need of an autopsy. We bought our coffees from a girl in her late teens, with blonde dreadlocks and a scowl for anyone without them.

"A latte, please," Norman ordered.

He turned to us, obviously preparing something, a mischievous delight ballooning in his face.

"What kinda milk?" the girl asked, a husky cruelty in her voice.

Norman's eyes widened.

"Breast, if possible," he said, eliciting from her a miraculous open-mouthed smile.

In her teeth, she didn't have a single filling.

"Whole," she confirmed.

Onstage, the keyboardist sits on the keys, bouncing along from the low frequencies to the high, his tailbone doing the dirty work. We watch from our table, and outside the window, the surreal product of the marijuana harvest continues to breathe. A teenager walks past and shows us his armpit. He's followed by a twentysomething woman who flashes her abnormally long and triple-pierced tongue. Norman begins drumming on the tabletop again.

"Delicious," Johanna says to the passing woman.

"Mmm-haaa-aaa," Norman laughs, embarrassed or not, I can't tell.

We're quiet for a while—four surf-gospel songs' worth of silence. The madness unspools around us like a solar system, but at this heavy table, I feel fixed. One of its legs. One of its screws. Johanna is fixed with me, and Norman trails after his own orbit as if on a dog sled. The weird music becomes commonplace, another footnote in the Encyclopedia Californnica.

I touch Johanna's hand under the table. It is warm, and a little wet. When we first dated, she confessed one of her most self-conscious crosses-to-bear was her sweaty palms. I think I may have made a joke about lubrication, something my dad would have said before he stopped saying much after my mom got sick. She looks at me, and in her eyes are the lives we've led. Collapsing legs, exposed screws, but a fucking beautiful tabletop somehow sustaining the weight of this bacchanalian meal. In the space between us that stops just short of Norman are my year living in Italy picking wine grapes and mopping cantina floors, my years in Alaska, a portion of which were homeless.

The restaurant where I had been working closed and the winter was coming up. I had to break into the apartment of a seasonal couple, some of the former restaurant's best customers. While these two spent their winter in a warmer place (Thailand), I commandeered their bedroom, bathroom, kitchen. I used the pots and pans of the people I used to serve—ham and cheese omelets for him, blueberry pancakes for her. Always coffee. I watered their plants and kept the place clean.

For Johanna the space contains the year she spent in Kenya working as a nun at a shelter for teenage prostitutes (the girls there would shoot drugs under their toenails because it was the last place they still had fresh veins); and her work as an au pair for a family in Israel. Their little boy fell in love with her. When she decided to return home to Sweden, the family locked her in (all the doors could be locked from the inside, she said), took her hostage. She had to sneak into the parents' room after they went to sleep, rummage through the drawers for the keys. She fled to the airport at 2:00 a.m. without any of her things. The customs agent ran his fingers through her hair, looking for miniature explosives.

And then: together in Chicago, this year . . . My mother's mortality still hangs like tar, even out here in California, in swaths of body paint and Charlie the Mechanic.

I don't let go of Johanna's hand. In this scene, teeming with life, immortal as cockroaches, I realize how much I am beginning to crave *boring*. How good *mundane* sounds. Because there's something familial in it!

I think about the purple handkerchief my mom would fold into her blouse pocket when she went to work. I think about that as the keyboardist falls from his stool and back-spins on the stage. I think Johanna and I were consciously trying to enjoy all of this—the music, the street scene, the sleeping in a tent and the dirty shower floors, the fields, The Mausoleum—in such a way knowing that this is as young as we are ever going to be, leaking our carelessness like blood.

In the keyboardist's back-spin is the nauseous bliss that dizziness can bestow only upon the preteen. This is the maneuver that ends their current song; that allows Johanna's hand to drop from mine, regaining its own space; that allows Norman to reassert himself.

"Yeah, I used to work these streets," he says, his voice snaking in from a distance, welling up from the bottom of some canyon in some desert where the wild daisies have just opened for their yellow, week-long lives.

"You did?" Johanna asks.

On the sidewalk, Norman would set up a barley twist French desk from the nineteenth century. He would sit behind it in a gilt Edwardian armchair, advertising his services.

"Faking antiques," he confirms, as the house band launches into a tongue-in-cheek 1950s doo-wop tune.

People would bring to him various items—jewelry, pottery, furniture, paintings, picture frames, lamps. For a fee, Norman altered the appearance of these items, allowing them a false age: antiques for the dupable. The consultation, wherein a payment plan and timeline were laid out, was free.

"You know," Norman explains, "sometimes people would have to drop things off and pick them up days later. It all depended: How long you hold it in the fire, how you rub duck shit into it, driving with the fan . . ."

His voice trails off as the band croons an irreverent "sh-bop, sh-bop" in unison. Johanna and I look at each other again. This time, we're both picturing Norman hunched over on the bank of some inland pond, shoveling duck shit into a plastic shopping bag . . . for his business.

The bald female singer throws her arms over her head and flits around the stage like a baby bee. A few customers raise their coffee mugs to her. She is evil and elvish. Like Norman. Like his old job.

"Didn't the police, um, have something to say to you about that?" Johanna asks him.

"Sure," he says. "They tend to do that. But this whole industry has to deal with that as a part. You can't have it both ways, though people tried. I mean, even Julia Child was a sexual omnivore. Mm-haa-aaa."

"Really?" I ask.

"Dude," Norman shrugs.

"You have balls," Johanna says.

"Wanda has the balls," he counters. "But we have to face the fear of being introduced to something else."

Behind us, at the bar, the sound of glass breaking, the blonde dreadlocked girl screaming, "Shit!"

Unmiked, she's still louder than the band.

Norman turns to me.

"This fear, dude," he says. "Ask your mother. It's all this twice-cooked Buddhist shit. The reality is: our generation has long been preparing for death."

I think of my mom's purple handkerchief, folded neatly into a triangle or diamond. I think of her folding it.

Johanna has this book on Color Theory. I remember her telling me that purple can signify romance and nostalgia, or gloom and frustration. I remember telling her that the author should make up his mind.

The music onstage swells, penetrates the back of my neck and stirs me to chills. I feel like we are waiting it out here, purgatory as sockhop, masked with a combat boot. Norman smooths his beard. Johanna tries to find my hand under the table again but only bumps along the iron legs, a dragonfly trying to find its way through a window screen.

My heart beats and I think of my mom kissing us goodbye as we left for California, our car sparsely packed, her body like chicken bones in a wool sack. I wonder about all that she put into that goodbye.

How heavily packed it was. I picture her waving in the side-mirror to a chorus of surf gospel—the waves that washed away God. She goes inside the house where my dad is watching a *Sopranos* rerun, pets Kodiak, and opens the refrigerator door. She does all the food shopping. In it is everything she expects.

The female singer rasps, "I'm just a pris'ner!" and Norman stops smoothing his beard.

"What do I know, dude?" he asks me, trying to diffuse some sort of unticking bomb, trying to make an antique of me. And I feel it: Johanna and I have been dropped off at Norman's old desk. Surely, we have already been faked.

I smile and shrug.

"I'm not sure," I say.

"I do know that in a past life, I was a walrus," he says.

I laugh; he confirms my impression of him as a formerly large mammal.

"Or Achilles," he continues, "bathing in some woman's bellybutton . . . Mmm-haa-aaa."

Johanna laughs, sips her coffee, lots of cream, lots of sugar. In her mug-bound decadence, I take a bit of refuge, try to find my old self, anything that's still genuine. I allow Weckman Farm, which seemed so overwhelming when we arrived, to render the rest of the world unmanageable. I decide to believe Thoreau for one more afternoon. From Norman, to Johanna, to the band, to the Slip 'n Slide Man, this town is a puzzle smashed, the pieces cut or burnt.

Like a flipbook of mug shots, I picture the faces of the picking crew, a strange anchor in this stranger sea. Crazy Jeff morphing into Gloria into Lance into Ruby into Bob into Hector into Charlie; shirtlessness merging with a windbreaker. Norman and Johanna smile at one another, slowly becoming friends. It's fun to watch.

We sip our coffee and talk of the farm, the female singer now riding the microphone stand like a hobbyhorse. Carved into The Verse's ceiling, grinning cherubs protest their imprisonment in plaster. The singer antagonizes the obese bassist with her steed, while the lead guitarist unlocks the gates of heaven with surfboard wax and a stolen credit card. As he rips his Pacific solo, Johanna and I finally, and vocally, flesh out our own rumors. We tell Norman some specifics of our time in Chicago, our journey to Weckman, the uncertainty of our lives after harvest season. We talk in order to regain something, even knowing that whatever it is has been forfeited for good.

"Reincarnation, dude," he says to us.

Johanna exhales out her nose.

"That's a joke."

"Oh," Johanna and I say in unison, but neither of us forces the laugh.

"There's no right decision," he continues. "We go along polishing the spoon, folding the napkins, folding the napkins, folding the napkins, then a flood of tears. Emotion is in formal repetitive experience, dude."

We go quiet.

Norman finally says something about how Tristan Tzara invented Dadaism after a brioche missed his mouth and went up his nose, "striking him with the nonsense of the world."

The song ends. The singer says something about Jesus reincarnated as a moth, always flitting toward the light of us fuck-ups. I think she's trying too hard. But she, too, has a load to carry, and she's doing it creatively.

The dusty drummer answers with a pound on his snare. He pops something into his mouth and bravely swallows it with bottled water.

"Repetitive experience," Norman repeats. "Wanda comes from three generations of tobacco farmers. And she carries it on. Repetitive experience."

He pauses. The band has yet to begin a new song.

Finally, he cracks his knuckles and says to the cherubs, "Confucius: boo! Aristotle: boo! They weren't even great assholes. Those guys could have learned from her. Wanda, I mean. They were looking for gold in the wrong room. They should have been on the farm . . . or in the kitchen."

He turns from the ceiling to us. We smile again, and drain our coffee. The music goes on as we step from The Verse, the guitar driving the life on the sidewalk, the sun farther west. The tabletop tarot cards hold silent, keeping their secrets to themselves, specimens on a slide, but without the microscope. As we walk toward Norman's Jeep, the warmth from our finished mugs still clings to our hands.

Eleven

NORMAN'S JEEP ROARS TO A STOP, a beast who, like a marijuana harvest, doesn't want to go quietly. Returning to Weckman Farm is like stepping from midday summer into a darker indoors. I have to blink a few times to see anything, this world draped in the cloak of purple afterimage. Everything is drastically mellow—the low drone of Charlie's one-seat tractor, Lance's voice rising from the fields in calm, disjointed syllables, Lady Wanda tucked into her envelope of mansion, probably rehearsing her next torch song.

Norman rolls from the driver's seat without vocal ceremony.

"See you later, dude," he calls thickly, the *dude* encompassing both Johanna and me.

Like rawhide, he's rollin'-rollin'-rollin' toward his lawnmower, an engineer who has found nirvana behind a humbler machine.

Johanna tells me she wishes that, from the beginning, she'd told everyone here she had a different name.

"But it's too late now," she says, "to be someone else entirely."

"We could always tell them that *Johanna* isn't your real name. That way your real self could be the fiction."

She takes my hand.

"It's something to consider," she says.

In the way she says it, she sounds like she's been cheated. At least for a harvest season, she could have been a broker consultant from Lodz. Does her accent really preach *Scandinavia* to the masses?

And as you know: because Johanna *isn't* her real name, and she *isn't* really Scandinavian, this section was written fill-in-the-blank style. After this, feel free to blindfold the prefix *meta*, give it its last cigarette, and fire away.

Johanna—still Johanna, always Johanna—surveys Weckman. No one has come from the fields to greet us, ask us about our trip from the frying pan to the fire. The food tent angles into the wind, convinces us it's going to capsize before righting itself. The same wind snakes through the Residents' Camp, as if from the depths of a bear cave, as if we'd now need headlamps to find our way among the tents, illuminate the true nature of hibernation as something that can kill us. Johanna squeezes my hand in a way that's either thankful or rueful.

"We should go home," she says.

My heart sinks, its blood draining.

"What do you mean?" I ask.

She sighs.

"What, babe?" I ask.

She's not looking at me, but at the fields, and the stink that they hold; the good people who give themselves over to sweat, reeking with season.

"I don't know," she says. "I feel like we're breaking the rules."

"Well, fuck the law, Johanna."

She drops my hand.

"I'm not talking about the law, and you know it. You know. It's like we're having jobs we can't even pronounce, you know? Like we're choosing a lifestyle we can't pronounce."

"Well, it's just for the season," I say, but know what she means. She means, we're homeless. I think also she means, though I hope not, and I'm unsure if I'd wholly agree, we're heartless.

"I think finally it's time for us to go. There are rules," she says.

I have to laugh now, a little.

"There are?" I ask.

She smiles now too, also just a little.

"Definitely," she says.

"So is going back to Chicago conforming to the rules?"

Her smile drops.

"Shit," she says. "You know, I don't really think so."

I nod.

"But it may be closer to the rules," she says.

Charlie's one-seat tractor shoots from Tractor Alley and tears across the volleyball court. Johanna and I decide not to decide for a few more days. Together, we walk toward the fields, and Charlie, even at all the good speed a one-seat tractor can muster, spots us and spins his wheel. He bellies up.

"'Bout time, brother," he says. "Some of us been pullin' double-duty. Like Wanda says, the work *will* get done, one way or another."

"Are you giving us shit, Charlie?" Johanna asks.

He smiles. His splotchy orange beard spreads like marmalade.

"Shit," he says. "We all get out in stages. Just glad you're back. How was town? The full scene, I'll bet."

We tell him about the Slip 'n Slide and the dice-juggling, the man with the beanless maracas, the squatting over the mirrors.

"Yep," Charlie says, his voice even raspier than usual. "The freaks and the geeks. These are our people."

He starts to spin the tractor away from us.

"Gotta get this shit to the Bat Cave," he says. "Meetchya at dinner. Watercress quiche, I think it's gonna be."

He steps on the gas. The tractor coughs into forward motion.

"Watercress fucking quiche," Johanna says, her vulgarity heading straight to my pants.

We kiss, impatiently, but we kiss.

BEFORE DINNER, still reveling in our day off, Johanna and I walk into the kitchen, where Alex, Emily, and Antonio are busy whipping, chopping, and scrambling, in search of some coffee. Our trip into town has left us exhausted, especially in the eyes.

Under the shed's blue roof, eight deep skillets sputter an egg and cream mixture on eight burners, eggplant lazes on the grill, the chest freezer stands open a crack like a coffin in a zombie movie, the commercial mixer pirouettes its paddle, and a walk-in refrigerator tries to keep its secrets.

The chefs nod to us.

"There," Alex says curtly, gesturing to the coffeemaker and its three-quarters-full pot.

"If you finish it, please make another," Emily says.

Antonio says nothing. He flips the eggplant slices, brushes them with an ancho chile spiced oil, and disappears into the walk-in.

Under these fluorescent lights, in the middle of this gleaming silver equipment, Alex and Emily lose their look of placid hippie chic, replaced by something vaguely militaristic. They strangle the handles of their whisks. In here, their features harden. In here, they know what has to be done. All malaria can be beaten. All great literature can be burned to start a cook fire. Only Antonio maintains a consistency. Both in and out of the kitchen, he shuffles the shuffle of someone who has been there, done that.

In the time Johanna and I have poured our cups of coffee, Antonio has been in and out of the walk-in three times. Each time, he emerges empty-handed. Alex and Emily say nothing. The fourth time Antonio starts for the walk-in, Johanna and I give in to our curiosity. We follow him, our coffee sloshing up over the lips of our cups, reddening our wrists with a sweet burn.

Peeking into the walk-in, we watch Antonio press his fifty-year-old paunch against a white bucket of vegetable stock. Amid the shelves, strewn with open-topped cardboard boxes of celery, carrot, yellow squash, buckets of pickling juice, olives, and oxtail stock (which I think has likely gone unused for the season), Antonio puffs marijuana from an apple. In an act common in restaurant kitchens, Antonio has fashioned a makeshift pipe from a partially hollowed-out Granny Smith. Part of me wishes he'd noticed our spying, said something goofy about keeping the doctor away, but alas . . .

He holds his lighter to the top and puffs from the side, passing the fruit to a set of much skinnier fingers. This second set of hands emerges from behind the stock buckets. We can see only up to the wiry wrists, decidedly female tendons poking through the gristle. Johanna and I sip our coffee and know these are the stringy wrists of a yoga instructor.

It is Robbi, Johanna's childhood friend, not with her giant man in Fort Bragg at all, but finding her off-duty refuge in a walk-in refrigerator, pulling weed from an apple. She steps from behind the buckets but still does not see us. She is wearing a baby blue jacket with a white fake-fur-lined collar. She passes the apple back to Antonio and leans into his neck. Her tall stork's body presses against his roundness, the pink tip of her tongue finding his ear.

Johanna and I look at each other. Antonio and Robbi? This is definitely a breaking of the rules. We will talk later about all of the secret lives at Weckman, about the trysts we never discovered, the conversations gone unheard. This cute, married speculation is something I will spare you.

Robbi mews something to Antonio. In her voice, hoarse from god-knows-how-long of hiding out in a refrigerator, the only word we can make out is *abundance*.

THAT NIGHT, at dinner, Bob inhales his quiche, and Hector's absence has us worried. Crazy Jeff and Gloria are gone too, but at least we know where they are—fighting the Squareheads (as Lady Wanda calls them) in Sacramento.

I listen to everyone talking, just stare at them as if in front of a bathroom mirror, shaving.

"What are you doing here?" I ask myself, but it isn't my voice. It's a caring voice, a voice maternal or paternal, one that is trying very hard to avoid saying the word *stupid*.

I listen to Charlie chastising Bob for his table manners.

"That's some abysmal shit, brother," he says, as Bob spews crumbs of egg custard back onto his paper plate.

I listen to Lance discussing the logistics and speed necessary in tomorrow's picking, Ruby answering his every utterance with something affirmative. I listen to Johanna biting her lip, trying her damnedest not to tell everyone about what we saw in the walk-in.

I think about Johanna's assessment of our lives; about some future home of ours filled with the luxury of thick bath towels and expensive dish soap, the middle-of-the-road holiness of a picket-fence mouse pad and a living room full of IKEA.

Sometimes I feel as if everything people say is holy. Other times, I feel as if I've heard it before. Tonight, our meal is draped in redundancy—Lance and Ruby tickling one another's hands on the picnic table bench; Bob and Charlie adopting their sidekick/leader roles; the usual absences; the food disappearing from our plates. I'm starting to feel antsy, as if trapped in a droning classroom, ready for the bell to ring. Tomorrow, we will pick, massage, cook, eat, talk, mow, and not move on. Or does the moving-on lie in the picking, massaging . . . ? I can't believe we still haven't figured these things out. Can't believe that we likely never will.

Bob, without meaning to, answers, "It's all a steaming pile of bullshit!"

He's telling Charlie about the "real" lack of security at Weckman Farm, doubting Hector's resolve.

"I mean, where is he?" Bob continues. "Where does he go?"

"His business, brother," Charlie says.

"We need some kind of rule here," Bob says, "otherwise . . ."

Lance pulls a strand of his hair from his mouth and counters.

"Shit, man, we're all here to escape that kinda shit . . . Come and go as you please, you know," he says.

"Oh, fucking child prodigy here," Bob says. "Little Boy Blue, boss of the fucking fields."

"Fuck you," Ruby pipes in a small voice, a mouse, microphoned.

She shuts everyone up. No one expected this from her. Her eyes harden. She threatens Bob with the most Medusa-like parts of herself. Lance touches her leg and her jaw unclenches. Johanna touches mine and I sigh. We finish dinner in silence, Bob sulking with his elbows on the table, Charlie staring at some silent thing hidden in the distant redwoods.

174

Twelve

I'M IN ANOTHER BACK SEAT. This time, it's in an Oldsmobile Cutlass Supreme, black exterior with plush maroon seats. One of those back-seat armrests that folds up and down. Thick like an ottoman. A king-size pillow-top bed for a Ken doll. I have no idea where this car came from. It seems to have slipped through the cosmos from the Oldsmobile afterlife, resurrected here on the Weckman Farm version of Earth to finish old silver-haired business. To deliver us—Norman at the wheel, Lance in the passenger seat, me in the back—to a local dispensary. We have a delivery to make, and I have managed to crash the party.

Out the window, the redwoods play their cards close to their chests as if in instruction. Norman is visibly nervous at the wheel—oddly straight-backed and oddly silent. He doesn't answer Lance's questions.

"Did Mom tell you to go this way?"

Norman leans his chin forward, handlessly mops his beard over his chest like a bushy windshield wiper. I think of Johanna busy massaging. She had to stay back today. With so many Pickers, I am far more dispensable, open to accept Norman's invitation.

"Dude," he urged this morning. "We could use one more body." With this, I was struck with a self-actualization at once exhilarating, depressing, and, thankfully, fleeting. For a few seconds, I really found myself, realized exactly who I am: *one more body.*

With it, we loaded, and I mean *loaded*, up the trunk of the Cutlass

Supreme with shoeboxes of pot, various strains (Trainwreck, Durban Poison, Northern Lights), and various box brands (Avia, Adidas, Stride Rite, Dexter). We carry several pounds' worth. We are the Payless Shoe Source of Reefer, a sneaker with smokable laces. We will not be undersold.

Though Lance assures me that the law is on our side, I can still feel my heart playing hopscotch in my chest. I start to miss Johanna.

"Legally speaking," Lance says breezily from the front seat, "we can transport eight ounces per patient served."

"That's good to know," I say, my palms beginning to become as slick as my wife's. *Contagious?* I wonder.

Norman looks to Lance with a *Yes, but* glance.

"That said," he continues, "if we're pulled over, we can be searched, and if we're searched—depending on the cop—we can be busted. The law isn't exactly explicit on the legality of selling to the dispensary."

"Which doesn't bother your mother," Norman says to Lance.

"Who's your mother?" I ask Lance.

"You know," he says. His voice is sheepish here, one of his secrets, though obvious, revealed.

And I do know, but it hadn't occurred to me before. Beneath the fat and the sequins, the ponderous, almost frightening breasts and day-glo eye shadow, Lady Wanda, in her authority and sensuality and quiet confidence, is Lance through and through.

"Lady Wanda," I say.

"Yup," Lance says.

"So that's why you run the fields," I say. "You're the boss's kid."

Lance turns and grins. Like a retired sheep, he's through being sheepish.

"Don't make me come back there," he says. "Besides, you need all the instructions you can get. Why do you think we take you on these errands?"

"The dashing good looks?" I ask.

"Because you can't pick for shit," Lance smiles. "Slow as molasses. Charlie, the old man, picks like four times as fast."

"Hey!" I say, laughing. I hadn't realized that this was my reputation here, my life a secret even from myself.

"We might as well wait for the fucking wind to blow the buds into the boxes," Lance says and begins miming my slowness with the scissors, opening and closing his hand like a half-frozen arthritic.

I tug the back of his hair and he laughs.

"Speedometer," Norman says to Lance.

Lance snaps to attention.

"Sorry," he says.

I can't get over this yet. "Really?" I ask, but neither answers.

Lance's job as shotgun passenger is to watch Norman's speed, to make sure he doesn't exceed the limit. With our trunk full, Norman drives by the textbook.

We pull up to the dispensary, which looks like an unmarked Starbucks, a small, unassuming, malformed structure that seems excised from some former strip mall, the lone holdout, the headstone testament to now-defunct pawn shops and hair salons, and park in the tiny lot. Old ghostly sales of guns and shampoo hang gauzy in the air. It looks quiet inside. Very few customers. Of course, such places are not open to the public but serve patients with a doctor's written authorization and a buzzer-operated front door. Some dispensaries act as underground social clubs, holding yoga classes, potluck dinners, movie nights, reading groups, and counseling sessions for terminal patients, requiring the participating patients to join before they can purchase the product.

Gathering the shoeboxes from the trunk, Lance leads Norman and me to the locked front door where he presses the small buzzer. The door, shaded with orange miniblinds, swings inward, and I get the feeling we're on hidden camera.

"Come in," a soft, feeble voice intones.

This is Wexler, proprietor of Alternative MedCare (both names slightly altered, duck shit rubbed into them). He steps into the shadows of his shop with a quickness that belies his sixtysomething years and frail body covered in burn scars. A former pastry chef, Wexler, in the late 1980s, suffered third-degree burns on most of his body, decimating his nerves and rendering him partially paralyzed.

"I was addicted to painkillers before I got into this murdering business," he says, proudly showing me his display case. "This morning, I baked some really good murdering chocolate cake."

I wanted to ask him if his phrasing was social commentary, calling attention to the American popular entertainment practice of demonizing fucking while glorifying killing, but decided that this would be far less interesting than a simple vocal eccentricity, so I shut my murdering mouth.

I step toward the counter as Wexler takes the shoeboxes from my arms. His fingers and neck are long, his nose short, and his gray hair closely cropped, immaculately shaped. His burn scars hug his bare arms like old cornmeal crusted over. His thin horn-rimmed glasses give him the look of a man who lives out of a briefcase, a former wild-haired attorney finding conservatism in middle age. Timothy Bottoms's law student having outgrown *The Paper Chase* (a film Johanna and I took refuge in in Chicago, routinely drowning out my mother's coughing fits, quoting, "Mr. Hart, that is the most intelligent thing you've said all day!" Shit, we were cruel in our sadness, but that's my family . . .).

Across from the counter are six round coffee-shop tables and chairs. A mural of Moses and his followers adorns the wall, painted joints twined in their fingers, the desert through which they hike sprouting a wavy Golden Gate Bridge: the Old Testament crossbred with psychedelia and hometown pride. On the far wall opposite the front door, a red curtain hangs over a doorway, hiding a mysterious back room. I hear the sound of a ceiling fan but don't see one.

I watch as Wexler rounds the counter, kicking dirt from his blue suede shoes, and joins the various strains of marijuana and marijuana baked goods—cookies, brownies, peanut butter cups, truffles. Marijuana as green as the grass, marijuana as red as blood, purple pot, blue pot, pot that strays to yellow, pot that brags its brown. Wexler stands with his hands on his hips as if he should be wearing an apron, as if he is a horticulturally sound butcher, ready to slice a plant into parts. I want to ask for half a pound of stamen, a full rack of lateral root. I imagine customers fainting because they can't stand the sight of spattered soil.

On the wall behind him, old Black Panther pictures, a poster of Buddha rendered in graffiti art, a black-and-white photograph of a naked woman cartwheeling in a cow pasture, a mounted, defunct television, and a spherical red Chinese lamp, turned on and off with a golden rope.

Wexler quickly bends and removes the murdering cake from the display case, cuts a piece with a steak knife, and breaks it into four chunks with his long, scar-latticed fingers.

"Try," he instructs.

We do. The chocolate is bitter, Venezuelan, tempered with the sweet earthiness of marijuana pulverized in a coffee grinder.

"Cannabis flour," Wexler names the ground pot he uses to season his pastries. "I'm thinking of adding it to the inventory, selling it by the sack. For baking purposes. Cookies . . ."

His voice trails off as he bends again, retrieves from the unseen floor a microscope surely gleaned from a child's chemistry set, and a triple-beam balance. Lance and Wexler begin to go through the shoeboxes, weighing the medicine and taking turns inspecting it under the microscope.

Wexler squints into the eyepiece and says, "Good, good. No trace of rot, no murdering pests."

"Excellent," Lance says.

I feel good, some pride in my slow-as-molasses work.

Norman goes in and out, bringing the rest of the shoeboxes from the trunk. When he is finished, he roves silently among the empty tables, allowing Lance the authority to do business. Today, though decidedly unmuscular, Norman is the muscle.

"Look at this," Wexler continues. "Check out those lovely drops of resin. They glow!"

Together, Lance and Wexler weigh the buds. Since our crop is so plentiful and the scale is so small, this takes quite some time. Eventually, Norman and I plop onto the high-backed chairs and pretend we have hot mugs of coffee in front of us. Our index fingers hook the air. We listen to Wexler speak a series of numbers, a series that Lance repeats.

Eventually, Wexler says, "I'll get the cash. I can certainly use most of this, but I'll take it all, sell the rest on consignment."

As he moves his burned body toward the red-curtained doorway, a thin woman emerges from it with a paperback dangling from her hand.

"Lance!" she says like a sickly torch singer, her black hair graying at the roots and tips.

"Hi Barbara," Lance says.

Wexler disappears behind the curtain, and Barbara says to Lance, "Are we doing the Book of the Dead today?"

Lance turns to Norman.

"We have about an hour," Norman says, though I can't guess how he knows this since I don't think he's ever touched a wristwatch.

"Sounds good," Lance says.

I'm not sure what's going on.

"Let's go in the back," Barbara says, "where I can lie down."

Norman tells me: Lance helps people die. He reads to them, these terminal patients in their chaise lounges, air mattresses, blankets, their solarium behind the red curtain. Barbara is the only patient here today, stretching onto a recliner beneath a ceiling lined with skylights. The room is narrow and long, a hallway of receptacles on which to lie down. The walls hold no decorations except faded yellow paint and a few stereo speakers through which no sound presently pumps. Lance sits in a straight-backed wooden chair next to the recliner. Last month, he and Barbara finished *How to Succeed in Business Without Really Trying*.

"You should have seen how it inspired him," Barbara tells me, her fingernails straying to black as if they are the first part of her to go. "He's going to be some kind of CEO one day."

Somehow, I can see that perfectly.

"We'll see," Lance says, taking her smooth hand in his and turning to the middle of the Tibetan Book of the Dead, reading something about a four-headed snake crawling through the afterlife. After two pages, she is asleep.

Back in the Oldsmobile, I tell Lance about my mom, about the last year. In his silence, his listening, there is a depth of comfort and communion. He nods, his hair warm on his shoulders, his breath held. What I had mistaken for tiredness in his voice is patience, the weariness that comes with being old beyond your years, having seen, and accepted as beautiful, so much death. He exhales, heavy, releasing out the half-open passenger window the youngest of sighs, the weight of the aging world.

Thirteen

IT IS ILL-ADVISED to stroll aimlessly around Weckman Farm at night. I suspect this is true of most marijuana farms. Charlie the Mechanic fancies telling stories about the "Great bloodbats of the redwoods, brother. Suck yer neck limp as a rubber band."

I think of airborne rodent teeth traveling at considerable velocity and bite at my fingernails. But there are certainly worries more logical. After all, in darkness, I am a human shadow, easily mistaken for an intruder—government official, militiaman, neighborhood raider. There's a sniper about. An epileptic one. Waldo, Hector's graveyard-shift replacement, is somewhere up in the trees, staving off a fit with a mug of Blue People Oolong tea. I imagine his left index finger snaking the glass handle of his teacup, his right strung over a rifle's trigger. This does not for peace of mind make.

But I have to walk. My heart needs calming. Further, I already realize that Johanna and I will not be staying until the end of the harvest season. We already have the gasoline in our veins, the conversations about leaving the farm that can not be undone. Somehow, we've been branded flighty, the iron having left its mark on more than just our skins. I don't know where we're going to go after this, and it's not necessarily back to Chicago. Maybe we'll return to Taos, New Mexico, where we lived a couple years back, out of our tent, along the ski valley road for the summer, bathing in the frigid Rio Hondo River with environmentally friendly soap and shampoo, shitting in a pit toilet where the only paper was the Subway sandwich napkins that a neighboring squatter left as a courtesy and mark of his day job. These were the days before we upgraded to the Cimarron. Maybe we could get our old restaurant jobs back at the Sagebrush. Maybe we've lived that life already.

So I am compelled to wander the night-Weckman, I think, as a way of collecting goodbyes. Tonight, it recalls the lullaby of a children's book: *Goodbye redwoods, goodbye crops, goodbye food tent, goodbye sniper tower . . .* I wonder if, under Wexler's burn-scarred watch, Barbara still sleeps. If Wexler himself dozes behind the red curtain. I have to walk. Johanna is not happy about this. Now, she rests on her side in the Cimarron, hopefully rediscovering sleep. I had the dream again, of my mother drowning in a volcanic lahar, frozen into position, a Pompeii refugee exiled to Illinois. As always, natural disaster has quite a reach. Tonight has been nothing if not pyroclastic.

I woke with the typical cold sweats, something manic, but moribund, in my chest, and the need to walk the dream off as if it were a cramp. A good night's sleep remains a marathon's distance away.

"Please be careful," Johanna whispered as she retraced her steps back into a good dream—maybe the one she always has about canoeing in Sweden along the Kalix and Angesan Rivers, on the back of a benevolent roan cow.

Unzipping the tent tonight is the loudest thing in the world, the Residents' Camp draped in a chorus of snores. The nose whistle must be Bob. The grunting must be Charlie. The low, moony moans must be Lance and Ruby, finding, in sleep, the open spaces of each others' necks, and some dream-meadow lit up in lunar white.

I find the wind tonight only by walking. The air at this hour is an otherworldly brine, the moon pregnant with the Pacific and wetting its bed, the dampening sky rewriting the tide tables in fatigue and discomfort. Each star is a blossoming rash. I imagine the longhorns a few miles away, their snores not unlike Charlie's, their heads resting on each other's spines.

And beyond them, the matchstick cemetery, the dead so modest under this leaking moon. Tonight's light is one of outlines, the shapes of trees perfectly edged, but their middles murky. Tonight, like expensive linen, is lined with silver. Tonight is the optimist's wet dream. In it, a lone crow calls out to the lost murder, who do not answer, underlining its loneliness with beak-yellow highlighter.

I pass Hector's tent. It lies in place like a carcass. By the way the wind caves it in, I can tell that it's empty, its ribcage picked clean by the vultures. I wonder where he's gone tonight, envisioning a redeye shift as a soccer coach, a wayward and lengthy drive into an open-all-night Los Angeles, the push to make it to Mexico. Where does he go? I imagine the laminated postcard on his tent door, autographed divinely:

> *Dearest Hector,*
> *Best Wishes!*
> *The Virgen de G*

I turn from the tent and walk beyond the Residents' Camp, turning from the crops and toward the redwoods, standing like pillars on a plantation house for bloodbats and their caged birds. Across from the trees, Lady Wanda's mansion sits dark and quiet, a mere footnote at the bottom corner of this forested page.

The night, even in the trees, is blissfully mosquitoless, the insects likely having latched onto Hector, carried out of Weckman by the magnetism of his sweet blood. The redwoods rock slowly as if in genuflection to the night, creaking with history, haunted and antique. Norman did not have to rub duck shit into these to allow them the appearance of age.

I stand, one inch tall, at the bases of their trunks, roots thick as a pipeline, in a natural nighttime jail. The marijuana crops flitter in the distance, trying to sneak me the exit key. But tonight, I don't want to be sprung. Not just yet. I embrace these confines over sleep; their scariness has nothing to do with the death of my mother. There is no real grief in putting oneself in danger. *Goodbye grief . . .*

In these trees, their tops muddled in darkness and a soupy moon,

I listen for the cocking of Waldo's rifle. In these trees, I imagine the sound of a weapon clicking could be nothing but gentle. I tread lightly, listening. I hear only the wind. I wonder if Waldo has fallen asleep at his post.

Tomorrow is another day in the fields, one without Crazy Jeff's laughter and politicking, one without Gloria's one-word questions and confused affirmations. Tonight, they are somewhere in Sacramento—a city I've never seen but imagine diamonded with orange lights. For the two of them, it's another fight that both drains and refuels them. I think of this past year, our fleeing from Midwest to West, lopping off a prefix as if decapitating a stage in our lives. Strange, when the same thing sickens and heals us.

When they left, Gloria wore no homemade T-shirt, her former cleverness having dissolved into old prescription-drug cocktails. We have to wait here at least until they return. I feel old, or aged, but falsely so, as if Norman really had rubbed his duck shit into me, held me in the fire, dried me, like a string box of marijuana, with a floor fan set to medium. For Johanna and me at this point, whimsy has gone the way of Gloria's mind, having drowned in a suburban Chicago sump pump, seeded green into manicured lawns. What else can I do but handcuff myself to this melodrama as punishment, as, perhaps, protection. It is my wetlands, my glossy ibis, and I stand between it and the flock of tractors who want to turn the place into a megamall.

But the redwoods seem to have the power to resurrect whimsy, if not Gloria's mind, as do the marijuana crops and encampment of tents, the sleeping bodies inside breathing small contentments into larger eccentricities, all of us as plastic and immobile as Resusci-Annie, waiting for a drunken Bob to crack our sternums in the name of heroism. But here, if only on Weckman Farm, his imperfect mouth-to-mouth will surely allow us to live. Resuscitating the flawed requires a flawed resuscitator. Maybe I should write bumper stickers.

In all of our desires to escape—from alcoholism and Vietnam, AIDS and cancer—we find a collective empathy. Maybe this isn't whimsy per se, but it's something whimsical. In this, the fucking-up can fuck down. (Can't you just see that on the back of a Plymouth Voyager?)

I run my palm over a redwood trunk, dig my fingernails into its meat. In it, I find a wetness, old rain or sap, the moon's diesel. I breathe and hear behind me a snapping—not of a twig or of a gun shifting its bullet, but of a bottle cap twisting open. I'm sure of it. I hear a sipping sound, the wet smack of lips pulling from a glass mouthpiece, a swallow followed by a tired exhale.

Aaaaaaaahhhhhh . . .

I am nervous but oddly comforted, in a parental sort of way. Before he became the sad man standing over the blue wastebasket of his wife's hair, my father was the flamboyant *Aaaaaaaahhhhhh . . .* after a long sip of Diet Coke.

I want to call *Hello?* but don't. My voice freezes, my breath pumped cold and smoky from my lungs. Instead, in an act that calls equally on self-preservation and -destruction, I weave through the redwoods toward the sound. I half expect to see my father, thirty-five again, doing push-ups between the trees.

Soon, against the base of a medium redwood (which, for a cypress, would be size 10XL), I see a strange shape floating about three feet off the ground. In this light, or lack thereof, it appears to be a giant disembodied brain, something that broke from the oversized pickling jar of a 1950s B movie and hid out here, filtered through Gabriel García Márquez, on the outskirts of Weckman, protected by an epileptic sniper. Is this guilt made manifest? Some ghostly return of the Latin *contritus* ready to grind us into pieces, crush us with the weight of our own skewed decisions? If so, it looks pretty fucking small, not up to the task; I hope this isn't one of those sci-fi scenes wherein the beautiful siren, when approached by the lusty man, morphs into a larynx-ripping alien with a thirst for frontal lobes.

I squint, and the shape mutates into something less solid: a plume of sea foam escaping the moon and the ocean. I step closer, and the shape shifts once more. I can see now that it is a head of hair, and that it is Hector's. He's sitting against the base of a tree, sipping from what in outline appears to be an Erlenmeyer flask. This is a surprise.

"Hector?" I manage.

His hands fumble with the air between them. He loses his grip on the flask, then regains it. I think I can hear his heart stutter.

"Oh, fuck it," he cries, trying to scramble to his feet before settling again into a seated position. "You scared the shit outta me, man. My God . . ."

"Sorry. I couldn't sleep," I say.

I don't think he hears me yet, the blood beating in his ears.

"What are you doing out here?" he asks.

"I couldn't sleep."

"Yeah. Right," he says, his breath and his heart calming down. "Well, you're welcome to a slug of this."

He raises his bottle. It is Agavero, a tequila liqueur of sorts, infused with fermented damiana flower tea. I sit next to him, the girth of the redwood trunk more than enough to accommodate us, and three conversion vans besides. Hector exhales again, still in the process of regaining his internal peace. I'm shocked to find that the air around him is mosquitoless. The Agavero must be a repellant. But not to me. Not tonight.

I sip from the bottle this thick mixture of cactus and petal, running over my throat and into my belly, a desert snake slithering with satin skin. I exhale. Like the snake, I want to rattle. Hector begins telling me how the ancient Mayans in Mexico used the damiana flower as an aphrodisiac.

"They would smoke the flowers, man, and go, go, go," he says.

"Wow," I muster, my throat regaining its elasticity.

"Good shit, right?" Hector asks.

But he knows the answer. Anyway, since he can only see the outline of my head, I nod.

"You could find a lot of shit in New Orleans, man, but you couldn't find this," he says.

He raises the bottle and toasts the moon.

"You can't hide, you fat white fucker!" he shouts, and I wonder if anyone in the Residents' Camp wakes up. I know Johanna can sleep through anything. If she sleeps.

"New Orleans?" I ask.

"Yeah," Hector says, and takes another sip.

He passes the bottle to me. In the moonlight, the bottle is green-black, skinny at the top and flared into a sphere at the bottom. Tonight, in these trees, Hector has attached a siphon to the globe, and is sipping from the core. If he chooses to share this delicacy with me, I can not say no. I take another swig and feel poisoned, poisonous.

"That's the good thing about California," Hector continues. "You can find almost anything you can find in Mexico."

I cough agave sugar.

"Well, not everything," he clarifies, voice trailing.

"What were you doing in New Orleans?" I ask as soon as the Agavero loosens its grip on my throat.

Hector exhales. His breath tumbles over itself, balled-up lace in the cool, and the white of the moon.

"Livin' there, man," he says.

He exhales again, a shorter breath this time.

"I lived there," he says.

IT IS ILL-ADVISED to dwell on the bark patterns the redwood trunk has burned into Hector's forearms. They cycle his wrists, scribbled highways devoid of blood, a testament to the impressions, sometimes ditches, nature digs into us. More to the point, I'm getting drunk, and the struggle to see such patterns makes me nauseous. At any rate, I'm thankful to the cosmos for granting me this strange goodbye.

I picture Hector in his treetop perch, having scaled a rope ladder to get up there, this wooden fort, large enough only for a bar stool, a tattered movie poster of Russ Meyer's *Supervixens*, Hector's boom box. He tells me he listens to Dr. Judy on the radio, the advice show that duels between medicine and morality.

"Have you heard this shit, man?" Hector asks. "It's unbelievable."

The sniper station: just enough room for this, and the gun. Hector never had to shoot anybody. Not here. Never spotted a trespasser. In the sniper station, he reads all the bestsellers about lawyers and doctors and serial killers and detectives. He comes to his job ready to commit himself to plot mechanics—stationing his gun in the corner, sitting on his stool, putting his lunchbox on the floor, taking in the panorama, turning on the radio, pretuned to Dr. Judy dispensing bad relationship advice. He reads a paragraph, looks around, reads another paragraph, looks around, takes a bite of BLT, looks around . . .

He hoists the bottle of Agavero and talks about it. By *it*, I mean this:

Hector was one of those rooftop shadows the Hurricane Katrina relief helicopters passed over. He waved a soaked white sheet that twisted in on itself like a braid.

"Felt like I was waving a lead vest, man," he says, pulling from the bottle and passing it to me. Furthering the theme of unreliability, I don't think he really said that. It was probably more like (mumbled, shit-faced), *Goddamn motherfuckin' lead vest, motherfucker.* You can substitute similar translations from sobriety throughout. Remember, I was pretty wasted too by this point.

He waves a moth from his hair and says, "That's what they don't tell you. That everything was as heavy as shit."

As he says it, I can hear his voice thickening. Or maybe that's my ear. He nods, folds his fingers into what may be a prayer, and bobs them back and forth, fishing for God without a lure. The wind is cool and, as if we were candles, nearly blows us out.

He lost two daughters, six and eleven, and a wife who was threatening to leave him.

"She never got to do it," Hector says, his breath deflating in the air. He drowns it with another sip of Agavero.

He was going to community college, wanted to be a guidance counselor at a high school.

The wind curls among the tree trunks, carries with it the sound of a false piano, the smell of false roses. The electrons between us shut us out, close the door on an atomic orgy, ions passing into an opium coma. The littlest of things, having the time of their lives, abandon us. I pat Hector on the thigh, thick as the roots under us but not immune to uprooting. Hector pats me back with a great social worker's generosity.

"Lady Wanda found me in Phoenix," he says at last.

"What were you doing there?" I ask.

"Family," he says, "I have some family there. Distant family, but you know. And I stayed with them for a bit before moving to this refugee camp, set up in the Coliseum there."

He pauses, runs his index fingernail over the ridges in the Agavero bottle. The sound is that of chains being dragged over a tile floor. The stuff of ghost stories.

"All I took," Hector says, "was this white laundry basket. Plastic."

"Why a laundry basket?" I ask.

"It was what I kept my things in."

Phoenix, like many American cities, turned its gymnasiums and concert halls, fairgrounds and basements, into refugee camps for those displaced by Katrina. In these camps, people slept, and woke, and ate donated food; drank donated water, their sweat asserting itself more every day, children becoming restless, clothes getting dirtier. In these camps, people died for lack of medication and medical supplies—no insulin or IV drips, tetanus shots or Tylenol. People died of minor cuts that grew with infection.

The number of people who had yet no bid on a future reached approximately 1.4 million. Local people tried to give what they could, crowded the animal shelters, adopting dogs with names like Gumbo, Jambalaya, Beignet, Po'Boy. A culture dying. A language surviving in the names of its rescued pets.

Johanna and I had old friends in Phoenix who volunteered at the Coliseum. I wonder if Hector ever met Eva and Tom, but I don't want to bore him (or you) with such irrelevancies.

Much of the federal relief went to the restoration of New Orleans hotels and casinos, chemical plants, and (as we all know by now) upper-class, predominantly white neighborhoods, while Hector and many, many others waited for hours in lines to get into buildings with names like Sky Harbor and Superdome.

"We had to wait outside in the rain for like five hours, while they searched everybody," Hector says.

Inside, people staked out their places in chairs or on floors. The spaces against the walls were particularly sought after, where people sat and rocked, missing things like a glass of milk. Unlike Johanna and me, these folks were not granted the luxury of choosing to flee.

I picture Hector in Phoenix, in the Veterans' Memorial Coliseum, lying in a hallway crowded with survivors, a cavern that once hosted Bruce Springsteen concerts. I picture him deep in a sleeping bag against a dark and caged concession stand, its beer taps empty, popcorn machine unplugged. I picture him trying to find sleep amid the ghosts of his family, beneath a neon banner sign advertising Pepsi. It's been much more fun picturing him in his sniper tree.

"You can't even imagine the bathroom situation, man," Hector says, mustering a laugh.

"I hadn't even thought about that," I say.

"It's nothing to think about."

He swats an insect from his ear, feebly. The more Agavero he drinks, the more tolerant he becomes.

He says something about lying down there, this four-year-old kid stepping barefoot over him. I look up to these giant trees and the giant sky beyond it, and imagine a tiny bare foot in their place.

He hiccups on the liquor a little but doesn't make a sound, like he's hiccupping in a silent movie. At any moment, I expect Charlie Chaplin to descend from the treetops and fumble with a parachute, reminding us how hilarious and precarious all of this shit is.

It's too dark to see, but not dark enough to miss the Coliseum, how he struggles to sleep there. The rustle of the displaced and misplaced drops over him like leaves. Children pad the hallways, climb over arena seats. Local volunteers plastic-wrap a metal tray of white rice, refrigerate it for tomorrow's breakfast. One hundred and fifty women wait behind a velvet theater rope to see the ob-gyn nurse, on duty for another forty-five minutes. The next shift comes in for the night, taking the flashlights and key rings from those who are going home to empty apartments and houses full of families. These nights: no stage or light show, no rounds of applause. The encores are across the country, buried under water.

Into this arena, and many others like it, came the farm owners of the American West, hiring these former Louisianans as apple pickers in Washington, cannery workers in Alaska, snipers in California.

Hector exhales.

"Lady Wanda herself came in there recruiting. A lot of people running marijuana farms came in there, offering jobs . . . and not for shit pay, either. Without her, man . . ." he says, shrugs, shakes his head, unzips his neck with the back of his finger. "This industry helped so many Katrina victims, man. It's fucking generous."

He sets the Agavero bottle between his feet. The glass catches the moon, lights up like a crystal ball. In it, I see tomorrow's hangover, the nauseating cling of marijuana resin to my hands, Lance whistling orders a few rows beyond. I see Johanna massaging in a room I've never seen, and Hector putting together his rifle as if a toy, a hobby horse, a remote-controlled car, long since running autonomously, without a battery in the world. We sit.

In this silence, I realize how exhausted I've become, my mouth petalled with alcohol, a cactus wrung out. I think of the nearest small town—the music, the Maraca Man, the fish caricaturists and their children, this generation of happy refugees—and these farms that attract refugees of another sort.

"Oh," Hector says, breaking the silence like a bottleneck. But he doesn't go beyond this. This is the sound, an old writer friend of mine once said, that is at the center of all poetry and, therefore, should never appear in a poem.

I wonder about Johanna and me. About my family. About what is and what isn't inherent in us. Somewhere, beyond these trees, Lady Wanda's mansion lies dormant and dark, another gorilla sleeping on its feet. I remember the word Robbi whispered into Antonio's ear during their clandestine tryst in the walk-in refrigerator.

Abundance.

This place is full of it.

Hector, by my side, reaches once more for the bottle between his feet. The shit just keeps heaping itself on. Drunk, I lean my ear into

Hector's shoulder, giving him an awkward hug with my head. He's as sturdy as a menhir, warm with booze.

"Well, like they say . . ." he says.

I nod.

"So what's next?" I ask him, lifting my ear from his shoulder.

He holds up the bottle.

"Let's finish this little bit and head back to camp," he says. "I'm tired."

I picture his big empty tent. The Virgen whistling in the wind. I picture Johanna splayed diagonally across the floor of the Cimarron. I feel lucky for such pictures.

"I mean," I clarify, "where are you going to go from here? After the season?"

Somehow, I think his answer may help to inform mine.

Hector pulls from the bottle, tilting his head back grandly. I silently pray he will howl at the moon, give me an excuse to join him—two guys being stupidly, happily male. He just holds an upturned palm to the sky. The night lights dapple his arm with shadow, the redwood tops draped over him like vines.

"The moon, man," he says. "I'm motherfucking Neil Armstrong."

Fourteen

LADY WANDA STRETCHES to full height in her cream chaise lounge, stirring a tall glass of limeade with her index finger. She collects the suspended sugar from the sides of the glass beneath a silver-painted fingernail, which she then brings to her mouth, and continues.

"Yeah, I found Hector there," she says, referring to the refugee Coliseum in Phoenix, Arizona. "What's with all these questions?"

My pseudo-goodbye draw to Lady Wanda rests somewhere in the realm of the Earth Mother—something sensual and matronly and protective—something I hope will allow me an igneous intrusion of the heart, the sediment of amity. That, and my compulsion to get an exit interview.

Lady Wanda, mother of Lance, brings her legs under her, her body coming to attention and, possibly, concern. She's wearing red Arabian pants with pink feathers at the ankle cuffs, the genie Venus who broke out of her clamshell lamp. She sits cross-legged, sets her limeade on a glass end table with a dull ring, and begins scratching both knees. She is wary of my questions.

I begin rubbing my temples with the thumb and middle finger of my right hand, streaking my face with the sticky filth of the crop. I've become immune to the smell, the dirt running the creases of my palms like a map of apocalyptic rivers. Last night's Agavero still has its hooks in me, my head pounding, a hangover chill gripping my spine, though the air today is mild. I couldn't accommodate much breakfast today, or much lunch. Johanna had little sympathy for me this morning as I hunched at the front of our tent door like a gargoyle, choking back my insides.

And now Lady Wanda has turned the interrogation lamp from her face to mine. The world brightens a bit, and I have to squint to face it.

"I'm just fascinated with how things work," I say.

Johanna is somewhere in the belly of her mansion, massaging our crew members. Another day . . . One of the last.

I finished my four-bite lunch early—whole wheat couscous studded with dried cranberries and preserved celery—and ambushed Lady Wanda on her porch before my return to the fields, pulled like a tiny rebel ship into her Death Star orbit. Another day of itchy forearms, the tickle of the fan leaves, the sting of the stem, the juvenile cotton-candy mess pushing its brown way beneath my fingernails; becoming aware of the muscles in my hands, their tightness, the red rings the scissors leave around my fingers, the sweat, the chill, another day . . .

"It can be fascinating, it can be boring," Lady Wanda says, reaching again for her limeade. "But yeah, I found Hector there. Hell, honey, we're all a bunch of fun-loving sad-sacks, didn't ya know?"

She begins telling me of the constant struggle she has with the dispensaries, maintaining these business relationships in the face of, as she puts it, "the zealots who misinterpret the law, or try to make definitive what isn't."

One such problem arose when a nearby town passed a moratorium on such dispensaries, even though the ordinance already in effect stated that a customer/patient could not purchase medical marijuana without a written recommendation from a doctor.

"All of a sudden," Lady Wanda professes, "I couldn't do business with a guy I'd been doing business with for years. Too much heat. I had to look at other cities, other towns, ride on my name. My family's known here, honey."

She cracks her knuckles. It's a thick sound, like preserved celery breaking. She looks tired, but serene. I remember fighting the urge to kiss the backs of her cruller hands, afraid that once I started, I wouldn't be able to stop.

Because Lady Wanda's longtime business associate operated in a "moratorium town," the local council refused to reissue his business license. Even though this associate continues to operate "as he always has," Lady Wanda says, "he's still operating without a license."

As such, the town's council can go to court and force him to close his doors as a violator of municipal code.

"It's just one more thing," Lady Wanda says, "that's not so fascinating. I have to worry about irrigating the property, providing electricity and supplies, keeping my books, doing the payroll—some people wanna be paid in cash, some people in weed. It's always something. And then laws like this, whole towns like this. The spotlight can save us or ruin us."

She actually did say something like this, and if at this point it seems as if I'm belaboring the point, providing further, but similar, insight into the marijuana industry when this story has already moved on to the rhythm of goodbye, it's because I was reluctant to leave, though convinced it was the right thing to do; I was hanging on to anything I could, belaboring points and conversations and relationships, because that blind leap into the dark, that drive out of Weckman Farm, that entrance onto some interstate with its Burger King and Flying J and Super 8 Motel billboards, seemed as daunting as death or birth, or anything with the prefix re-. There was something safe and soporific in Weckman, and in extending my goodbyes as long as they would run, without officially calling them goodbyes. In belaboring, here, is a measure of truth, though again, filtered through the aftereffects of overindulgence by starlight.

Lady Wanda pulls off her shoe—a ruby slipper of sorts—and along the top of her foot, I notice an all-green tattoo of a palm tree, a naked woman with the head of a cow swinging from its fronds with her head thrown back (some postmodern depiction of the goddess Hathor?). She scratches her cracked heel, replaces the shoe, and continues.

She tells me that this one particular dispensary associate "cooks" his marijuana into variously flavored lollipops for those patients whose illnesses prevent them from smoking. He uncovered this form of ingestion because he is sick himself—one of the many caregivers who doubles as a patient.

"He used to be on federal aid—disability," Lady Wanda says, "and now he's not. He's active, running a business. Giving back. That's what we do in this industry. We're only trying to help people. Fight to help. So many of us currently employ people who used to have homes in New Orleans. We just have to face legal battles to do it."

She sighs and sips from her glass. I imagine the cow-headed woman beneath her shoe, howling in a multispecial ecstasy. In the distance, a few crew members scatter from the picnic tables into the fields. The march of the laborers. Of the belabored. I expect soon to be dismissed to my cutting, which is, today, an afterthought. It's warm today, and, as Lady Wanda says, "the blood wants to work."

I imagine Hector up in the trees. The world that we all walk on so far below him—shadows and laboring ants. The winds up there, to him, must seem like nothing but soft blessings. Warm bread.

Lady Wanda hugs herself and swallows another draw of limeade. I picture her in her midnight blue evening gown, crooning "Eve of Destruction." She strikes me as the type of person who, in the aftermath of Armageddon, would grow six additional arms, would be responsible for repopulating the earth.

"What about you?" I ask her.

"What about me what, honey?"

I rub my palms together, marijuana dirt snakes coming together, rolling toward my thumbs.

"How did you ever get into this?"

She dismisses me with a wave of her hand and the creaking canvas of the chaise lounge. She bunches her face. She answers me quickly, and without much detail. Lady Wanda comes from a long line of tobacco farmers. Her father had bony elbows. Her mother, a full face. Lady Wanda was a girl who discovered lipstick early, was married. Her husband, a native Californian named Roy, worked for her parents on their farm. His great-great-grandfather came to California, prospecting for gold. Roy also had bony elbows, and thick tendons that protruded from his neck. Two years into their marriage, he became a heroin addict, grew a moustache and a patchy brown beard, died of AIDS, and introduced her to the virtues of medical marijuana.

"My parents were full of sympathy," Lady Wanda says. "They never pointed a finger at anyone. They began growing a small crop of pot to help Roy through it. It was the only . . ."

She pauses, sighs, looks up, watches a cloud break apart over her.

"So," she says in her best schoolmarm voice, "it's best to be sober as a judge. Like me. Sometimes, though, I have to sample my product."

She narrows her eyes and smiles, reaches with her chin toward the fields where the majority of the crew members are rejoining their clippers. This is her silent *Go, get the fuck out of here*, the gesture full of understanding, but honeyless. Our interview is over.

I stand on her porch, survey the fields below. They look like the ocean as seen from an observation deck. After weeks of sleeping on the ground, it's strange to be at such an artificial height—pillared and wooden. It's all I can do to step down.

"Thanks," I say to Lady Wanda.

"Mm-hmm," she says, her throat fluttering with limeade. "It's the meaning of work."

I'M BACK IN the fields, sweat at my collar, the middle of my back, the edges of my sleeves. I sneeze, listen to Lance's low instructions, Charlie the Mechanic's electrical wheeze, the swishing mediation of Bob's windbreaker, the quiet steps of Ruby's canvas shoes on soil. I pick marijuana buds from their branches, flick a wayward seed to the sky. The leaves fall away like hair clippings. The clippers creak, the blades of the scissors come together, a metal kiss over smokable medicine. In the fields of Weckman Farm, it's business as usual. Outside these fields, not so. Overhead, a massive flock of birds tears across the sky, a tangle of black outlines. There must be a thousand of them. One of them must be the matriarch.

A YELLOW LINCOLN Continental taxicab drops Crazy Jeff on an unmarked dirt road, two and a half miles from the entrance to Weckman Farm. He stands, kicking a jagged green bottleneck, severed from its bottle, along the side of the road.

At Crazy Jeff's feet rests a blue duffel bag with black straps. It is half-packed, the luggage tags left blank, nameless, without address. To this bag, and to Crazy Jeff's red T-shirt, Sacramento still clings. The bag's empty center appears deflated, underfed.

There's little wind in the redwoods today, the treetops barely whispering against one another, eliciting the kind of sound you don't notice until it stops. Like crickets. Like a friend breathing.

A minute later, not with his riding lawnmower but with a green and white sports model golf cart, Norman meets him. Picks him up. The way Crazy Jeff steps aboard indicates something—anxiety perhaps, or an unearned peace. He steps with weighted ankles and weightless arms, a finch with perfectly good wings, its feet caught in cement. Norman, thick-lidded, easy, takes his foot from the brake before Jeff is fully seated. Their heads bounce from their headrests in unison.

They say little, but do a lot of nodding. Not even the redwoods hear Crazy Jeff laugh. What little wind there is flattens Norman's beard to his chest, stirs a tendril of Crazy Jeff's hair. He holds the duffel bag on his lap, the soft clothes inside cushioning his shaving razor, black travel hairdryer, small bottle of bright green mouthwash.

He wears leather sandals with Velcro straps and stares at his feet. As a child, he always thought ill of men in sandals—it was something indecent and decadent, careless and complacent. Something his father said, maybe . . . Now, he is one of them, trying to divine his fortune from the lines of dirt on his feet.

Norman offers no advice but drives with a strange and comforting rhythm, as if the golf cart were a drum. Gloria is not with them.

In Crazy Jeff's head are equations: formulas he hasn't thought of in decades—the Pythagorean theorem, $y = mx + b$. The impossible stuff of his childhood. Problems he can't solve. He looks about. The redwoods stand, a few broken branches, stripped to bark and charred looking. The world to him appears as if under water. As if the ocean were a yellow tea and the sun were impossible. He wishes for the four hundredth time today that he wasn't sick. That health could be divined if only he carried the right number, borrowed the proper amount. That death could be swallowed up in a sloping line, kept captive at the bottom of a parabola, solved. On a sheet of graph paper, solved. Equations . . .

Norman's hands are steady on the wheel, and the golf cart bumps along as if the earth were a wooden track.

Everything rots, Norman wants to say, but doesn't.

He's thinking of equations, too. Tender ones. The redwoods watch them pass, their enormous trunks still. Jeff watches the trees, vibrating with the golf cart's engine, the rocky soil.

Forever, he thinks, is so much longer to them.

JOHANNA'S DAY ENDS EARLY, with plenty of light left in the sky. I join her an hour later, the late afternoon the color of potting clay. We watch with a few others as Jeff and Norman pull up in the golf cart, park against the stand of plants closest to the Sofa Room. Norman cuts the engine, but we can't hear it die.

From behind us, the German Shepherd emerges, walking quickly, covering ground, his strides giant. He has pushed the sleeves of his blue duck-hunter's coat to his elbows, the tight cuffs forcing the blood to his hands. His fingers appear abnormally red and about to burst. I remember reading about early American settlers, trappers and explorers: how they would bleed their horses and mix the blood with salt, preserving it; how they would cut the stuff into square cakes and save them for desperate eating when other food was scarce. The Shepherd's hands look full enough to feed the entire crew. Pounding the earth with his feet, making his way toward Crazy Jeff and Norman, he appears nothing if not nutritious.

With these swollen fingers extended before him, he approaches Norman first, then Crazy Jeff. He touches both on their shoulders, suspended between the two of them like Lady Wanda's volleyball net. For the first time, he looks like a doctor.

Johanna paces as they confer. A strand of her hair blows against my face. I shake it away, scratch, and then try to find it again. Her hands are hot, sweaty. She's anticipating something. Since we left Chicago, it seems as if she's been anticipating something, though I only first sense this now. Suddenly, I can't believe that I am a husband; have been for years.

Crazy Jeff drops his head and the Shepherd follows suit. Norman, for balance, looks up to the sky.

"Oh, fuck," we hear Lance say, the words carrying a panic, as if he's in a car he knows he can't stop before it hits the deer.

He swallows, returns his teeth to his bottom lip and chews. Ruby curls her mouth like a mute wolf, staring confused into some invisible sun, trying to uncover the source of its brightness.

"Matter of time, brother," Charlie says to Lance, his voice surprisingly smooth.

Lance pulls from Charlie and again says, "Fuck."

The deer is dead. The car is totaled. Somehow, we're still alive.

The Shepherd and Crazy Jeff continue to hang their heads as Norman looks skyward, his hands on his hips. He says something that makes them laugh, but we can't hear that either.

IN A SACRAMENTO BOARDROOM, a man in a solid black tie leans forward into a microphone, his thin fingers wrapping the edges of the podium. The light is bright, its fluorescence reflecting from the spray tightening his hair. He wears glasses that keep sliding to the bridge of his nose, his Adam's apple rising and falling. He snorts, suffering from some allergy, a simple gold wedding band on his finger. He speaks out against marijuana, medical or otherwise, uses phrases like *social decay* and *moral imperative* and *take control*. His voice shakes a little, and so does the white sheet of paper in his hand—his carefully prepared outline.

He is not without his pathos, Gloria thinks.

She sits collapsed in her wheelchair, a white cardigan sweater buttoned over her T-shirt of protest. The sweater's stitches are loose, big-eyed. It can't keep out the air. At this point, for Gloria, any air conditioning is too much. She listens to the man talk, his words jumbling together, riding their nonsense to the corkboard ceiling. She feels the ache in her back, the static at the back of her throat. She is nervous, but she doesn't know why.

COME EVENING, in the Sofa Room, under the bellies of all those Buddhas, Crazy Jeff tells us, "She was coughing so much more than usual. But even that didn't seem *un*usual, you know?"

We all huddle around him.

Charlie says, "Nothin' ya coulda done, brother."

Johanna chews her hair. I think about Chicago—the dirty snow, the traffic, the radio stations. I try to picture these people there and can not do it.

"Yeah," Jeff says, his cysts lying dormant at his ears. "Yes."

AFTER THREE AND a half hours, the Sacramento meeting adjourns for lunch. Crazy Jeff grips the hard rubber push-handles of Gloria's wheelchair. The man who just spoke out against medical marijuana smiles at them, politely gives them the right-of-way. The sound of folding chairs refolding echoes behind them.

They return to their motel room. Orange and green bedspreads. Yellow cotton blankets. Clean white sheets. A small color television mounted on the wall. An open closet with the hangers that attach to their plastic moldings like nailheads. Over the bed, a mauve-framed print of a wheatfield. The story of the interstate billboard made manifest, its promises of rest and relief fulfilled. Gloria eats one banana, drinks half a bottle of skim milk. Her throat feels like a failing mechanism, rolls the food instead of swallowing it. But it's felt this way before.

Crazy Jeff steps into the bathroom and turns on the light. It's one of those lights that automatically ignite the fan. Crazy Jeff hates that. This one is particularly loud. He unwraps the brittle complementary soap from its paper packing. It is pale peach. It cracks into four pieces. He takes the least jagged of these and soaps his hands under warm water, washes his face. The soap leaves its grease on his skin. As he tries to wash it away, rinsing and rinsing from the faucet, Gloria falls asleep on the bed to the History Channel—something about Nostradamus and the calm underbelly of Armageddon.

Over the drone of the fan, Crazy Jeff can hear the narrator say something about the 1500s and an apothecary. From here, he can see the night stand, but not the bed. The digital clock spews its red light. The wheat is frozen on the wall. Another meeting convenes in forty-five minutes. He bends again to the running faucet, but the water has not gotten any warmer.

"SHE WAS DEAD before the next meeting convened," Jeff says. "Probably while I was still in the bathroom, but I just thought she was sleeping. I didn't think right away to check for her breath. I thought, Just let her sleep, you know, just let her . . ."

He slumps on the sofa in Gloria's old spot, her drool stains on the cushion having outlasted her. I want to ask him about her body. I want to know who took her, who claimed her, where she is now. Though I heard her utter only a few words, and never directly to me, I feel Gloria was my friend. I know all about curing marijuana in a string box, but I don't know if, or where, she's buried. I have no idea where her body is.

I want to ask him about the probable trip to the emergency room, about the official pronouncement. I want to know how the German Shepherd knew before the rest of us. Perhaps he has connections to a Sacramento hospital. I wonder if Gloria has been buried or burned; if some never-mentioned brother came to take her. I wait for someone else to ask. I look around the Sofa Room at everyone's faces. They look as if blank slates that have been carved into—funereal jack o' lanterns. No one asks. No one is going to ask. I don't ask. Apparently, Gloria should die as she lived—as a mystery.

As Crazy Jeff tells us of his journey back to Weckman, slowly moving the silence around in his mouth like a gumball, I turn to Johanna. I see Chicago in her eyes, its shadows, tall buildings, the same alt-rock radio station we would listen to in rush-hour traffic, all crops long since plowed under, hidden beneath the earth. How, during the commercials, we would switch to the classic rock station—some Led Zep, Jethro Tull carrying us through the construction site, the Sears Tower, the stuff of childhood hometown pride, of *tallests*, disappearing into the city-murk behind us. I see the tired revelation that escape is a lie—impossible under the covers of family. In her eyes, I see all the paperbacks we have yet to read, the arguments we will have about what to cook for dinner, the beautiful lawns under which we will lay our parents, the difference between *hometown* and *birthplace*.

This Sofa Room is a wonderful room to move beyond. Outside, the crops gather moonlight, sustenance, dress themselves in the disguise of the prairie, the bog, the dregs of the Midwest and the field mice who dream there.

Crazy Jeff wipes his eyes and manages a soft laugh. In it is the stuff of prayer.

"And here we are," he says, rubbing his cysts, not to stifle, but to gather power, electricity. Inside him is surely the phrase he repeated upon our arrival here, the phrase that packed the hilarity of faux non-sense and sent him into hysterics. Surely, he wants to say it—*There's nothing more physical than physics*—but he holds back, allows us to consider the decorations in the room, the bellies of the Buddhas and all the food responsible for them.

I rake my fingernails along the back of Johanna's hand, and she says, "Spellbound."

She refers to that cameo seductress in the Hitchcock film, one of our favorites, in an early scene that fills the camera and is then, very quickly, forgotten.

In spite of everything, tomorrow we pick. To Lady Wanda, the day off is not something actual but a state of mind. Crazy Jeff is trying to organize something tomorrow night for Gloria—a tribute or service or sendoff. I imagine a sad collection of fireworks, muted colors, various blues. I hope we're not expected to speak.

Charlie slumps against the wall next to Lance, and Lance seems to catch him. Charlie, for all his accumulated experience—Vietnam, alcoholism, that mythical oil rig in Alaska—relies on Lance for support. And Charlie must be coming to terms with that. Strength is easy; it's having been broken and poorly reassembled that's hard. Charlie looks at Crazy Jeff and the two of them seem to share this thought, exhausted, but comfortable.

Outside, the winds rinse the Sofa Room's doorway, a wild howl snaking the tents, the crops, the slabs in the bloomery.

THE NEXT NIGHT, after work, hands washed as best we can, we gather to Hector's tent with candles. This is Lady Wanda's doing: old candelabra candles, skinny and white, stuck into small gold cups with their own wax. We each hold one like ancient stunned porters, newly woke, in nightcaps and pajama bottoms. The moon renders the earth to its bones.

The crops slush against one another in the dark wind. The stars are out tonight, watching. We stare into the bottomless laminated eyes of the Virgen de Guadalupe, Hector's taliswoman against Katrina and his own dead family, and now ours against the silencing of Gloria. This sort of weather, this mystery upon which we are compelled to force logic.

For minutes, nobody says anything. Johanna holds her candle under her chin, so close I wonder how she doesn't burn. Superwoman. Ruby holds to Lance, their flames in their outside hands. Bob and Charlie stand shoulder-to-shoulder, coretirees after a lifetime of hard communal duty. In spite of the wind, Bob's windbreaker tonight holds its tongue. The Shepherd stands, arms crossed piratewise over his large chest, the candle cup in his right hand, resting on his left shoulder like some spirit parrot.

"I remember when she was well enough," Lady Wanda says, her arms at her sides. "When she was fast."

Crazy Jeff clears his throat. Subterfuge.

Hector looks from the sooty eyes of the Virgen to those of the moon, taking aim. His forehead, a damp bark.

I wonder if Waldo can see us from the trees. The intricacies of our grieving, the hands held, the unheld hands.

The candle flames illuminate all of this tent canvas, our neighborhood, the Residents' Camp glowing, a topaz underwater, the scales of some warm-blooded fish. And behind us, the night crop oranged, waiting to be groomed, the deep breaths of all the people we serve—those who live and die with our help, die nonetheless.

Fifteen

THAT NIGHT, in the Cimarron, I have my mother's dream. And if you think this may be a rewrite of an account my mother wrote on a 1959 Underwood-Olivetti Lettera-22 typewriter, and I found many years later in a hutch drawer where I was snooping around while pretending to dust the furniture for my seventy-five-cent allowance, you're right. And if you think this doesn't make me nervous, you're wrong.

It's a warm day. Spring. April in smell alone. The sidewalks warm, feet newly sandaled, the sky without threat. Friends. In our skirts and ponytails—one with thick glasses, black frames, one whose mother let her wear blush for the first time, her heart nervous with it, afraid for what the extra red may bring her, crossing some kind of line where there were no nets to catch us. I can't remember their names. Struggle to make out which one must be me. Plaid skirts, thin socks, bags slung over our shoulders filled with school books, the stuff of science and spelling held aloft by our bodies, not strong, but young enough to dismiss the weight. We are light.

Through the maples, the breeze, sun, the leaves fresh green, that luminous green of prepubescent olive oil, and in it, flowers, white ones carrying cherry, orange, honey. Spring, and walking home from school with your friends—it's you now—bodies young enough to welcome the weather and its waking-up. The mob of grass shuddering, some wild shag carpet, begging to be pulled by the roots, thrown into the air as an offering.

Open your coat to prevent the perspiration from building. The collar at your neck going damp for the first time this year. Into the spaces at the sleeves, the breeze rushes, heavy with sap.

Your house, white with a distended window next to the front door. A leaf drops and you think this is not supposed to happen in spring. Your friends continue, one of them skipping, one of them calling your name, her hand high in the air, fingers stretching as if feathers drying off. Your house. Your mother's car in the driveway, not blue, not gray, the roof covered with green leaves, the things that should be living now, not dying. But the breeze has become a wind.

So strange to see this car. The crabapple tree at its front bumper evicting its petals. They come to rest on the headlights. Strange. She should be at work. Your mother should be at work. She's always had a full-time job, the thing that causes the other neighborhood wives to turn down their eyes when speaking to her, wrinkle their lips at the corners, allows them to feel sad and lucky in their costume jewelry.

At the curb, white, your aunt's car, white, petal-less, leafless, the windshield so clean it looks as if you can stick your hand through it, straight to the driver's-side headrest. Strange. Your mother and Aunt Karen do not talk. Stopped talking months ago—something about a bounced check and your grandmother's verbal, but unwritten, promise. Something your mother has told you, time and time again, is an adult conversation. Why would Aunt Karen be here? In spring?

Though your friends are now long out of earshot, mere specks on the sidewalk ahead, you say, Goodbye, aloud. You walk up the concrete steps, count them to yourself—one, two, three, four, five, six—and snake your fingers through the black steel of the door handle. Slow. As the door opens, the stench of matzo ball soup burning onto the bottom of the stockpot, scorched fat and wet meal, carrots as soft as cotton. In your stomach, feathers, an egg cracking, the first fluttering of unworkable wings.

Step inside, the beige carpeted stairs that lead up from the foyer to the kitchen, draped in a rigid plastic to prevent staining, the sin of dirty shoes. In the den, the piano that no one plays holds a vase of yellow carnations. Low voices, then no voices. Feet in black stockings stepping quickly over carpeting. Your mother. Black teased hair, sprayed stiff, thick-lensed glasses, a developing hunch, going blind in her left eye, your mother. Soon, it will be glass, but you don't know that. The shaking of her voice. The people standing behind her. Your two aunts. Your sister, Heather. Hands at their sides. Faceless. Hands at their sides.

Heather turning away, facing the carnations, then turning away from those. Nowhere to look, but look. Burnt soup. Shredded chicken thighs treading broth, black flakes lifting from the pot's bottom. Coins of yellow fat. The kitchen television turned off. Your mother with her reaching hand, the ring that your grandmother hid under her tongue for days. The infection that turned her mouth black. The ring from Poland, the opal filthy, unable to phosphoresce.

The pink loveseat in the den, the black and white photos in frames, the piano. Sitting there, you're sitting there. Your mother is speaking, her lipstick so red, her mouth a rubber band stretching and rebounding. Her face so caked in clay. A puppet. A performance. The real speaking after the rehearsal. To you. Speaking to you. She is leading to something else. The gemstone so small on her finger. The gold so dirty it looks brown. You are so impatient to hear, but you don't want to hear. The world, newly sandaled, so unprepared for an unseasonable cold.

Your mother is trying so hard. You think to punch her in the face, wonder about her taking to a broken nose, a fat lip. Your fingernails find the meat of your palms. Your friend, not the one who skipped or held up her hand, but the one who spoke your name, this is who your mother is talking about. Your friend, Linda. Her name in your mother's mouth sounds unwieldy, too much food for the teeth to bear. Your mother is trying so hard to relate all of these words to Linda, to the death last year of Linda's mother. Your mother says the word learned . . . when Linda learned of her mother's death . . . as if it were a subject she could study for, test well on. You forget about punching her, forget about all things swollen. Your mother's voice trips, falls down the plastic stairs. She manages. She tells you your father went to work this morning—his suit, his crooked teeth—he went to work this morning, she manages. With another man. A partner? A potential customer? He sells used cars, your father. He brushes his hair every twenty minutes. Your father. He went to work this morning in his suit with another man and there was an accident. An accident, and this other man was in the hospital.

This other man you don't want to hear about, his name is Artie. A cute oil painting, you think, an adorable, babyish sculpture: Artie. In coming grief, there is this inevitability of the joke. You're the youngest child. Jokes are your responsibility. A lack of care about this sculpture's injuries, however serious. When you speak, you speak deep, watery deep, your voice the penny tossed into the pool, falling to the bottom, the coupling of copper and concrete, the echo of a chlorinated choke.

"What about Dad?"

Your mother's eyes close, through the lashes, burgeoning salts. Her voice a vase cracking in the freezer. A cold break. On the wall behind her, the airbrushed portraits of you and Heather, Heather six years older and blond, your face round, your dark hair, the frames that hold you to the wall painted gold, anchored with broad lamps to shine on your faces.

Your mother runs her palm over her throat as if smoothing down, the veins on the back of her hand greening in the lamplight. She can not avoid this. This is what has become of her in this house, the piano, the cars outside, the sidewalk, the leaves, the flowers, the grass, her makeup and hairspray, cotton blouses and house-slippers, adding up to this, this mathematic of cruelty, and an appetite that will never fully return. In the future, in restaurants, she will only order what you order. Even if it's not the orange roughy. Everything about her billowing with ash. She is forced.

You are twelve years old and your father is dead. The scream is yours but comes from out of this room, this house, down the block, the school you walked home from, surrounded by boys who never kissed you, chalkboards filled with equals signs. Comes from out there, where you still walk with him past the playground. The woodchips. The swings. The slide. Where you go with him to visit your grandmother the next town over where she lives with his sister, your Aunt Lynn. His teeth yellow and smiling as he drives. So carefully. Always balls bouncing into the street, a jump rope hanging from a tree limb. The leaves falling like graduation caps, diamond and tasseled.

At Aunt Lynn's, while he whispers in the kitchen his verbal practical jokes, everyone laughing, faces red, you play with the dog, the golden retriever he named Electricity—the one your mother would never let you have. Never a dog in the house. Every Sunday, just the two of you. His stories of his childhood, how he would strip wires, rerig the doorbell to shock his sister's suitors. Sundays. Meeting him at the bottom of the plastic stairs where his shoes are already on and tied.

Weekdays, watching out the window for his coming home. Every day, he would drive a different car home from the dealership, so you could never guess when it was him, always, coming up the street, the surprise. One Wednesday, a lime green station wagon with wood trim. You liked that one. You remember this. You liked that one.

So tall with long arms. In your flight down the stairs, something of the sparrow and the sail, how you feel so cosmic, oceanic in the spread of his arms. The orange sweat stains of his undershirt hidden beneath his jacket. But you know they're there. You've seen them so many times.

The pictures of you and your sister on the wall. Airbrushed, as he lifts you, your legs heavy with gravity. His brown-brimmed hat, alpine on his head. This lean, small-waisted giant, smelling of spicy mustard sandwiches and motor oil. Blue eyes like dimes, brown hair, olive skin greased with evening. You have his hair. You wish you had his eyes.

How he stops for every pulled-over car—jumper cables, tow-rope, jack. How you watch from the back seat while your mother sighs up front, exasperated as he jacks. They, again, are going to be late. How he sleeps so little. How he is never home enough. The displacement, as your mother believes, of his charity.

The tightening of your throat as you prepare, maybe, to scream again. But don't. Don't. Don't look into your fat hand, feel the warmth of his. Don't smell his small dinner and auto grease and the astringent syrup of his blue aftershave. In don't is swiftness and safety. A place to belong. A retreat with a campfire and pianos that people play. Your mother's arms taking you into her chest, replacing something; your sister touching her forehead to your back, replacing something else. A normal breath. The breathing before this. Aunt Karen some freakish electron, moaning away like a ghost.

Your mother snuffing her eyes with her thumbs, Heather leading you upstairs, urging you to lie down. Some bed. More comfortable than ever. Did the dresser always have that mark? It looks like lightning. Did the blinds always hum like a refrigerator against the pane? Lying down. Springing up. Your bones being towed, that tow-rope, yellow, that yellow force. Your ribcage plucked, some blistering instrument. The good Samaritans of the world going invisible. You, for a second, want to be with your sister and your mother, scared in this room, scared here. The blur of the walls, their red and white paper, fathering a kind of slaughter, the stitches of the red carpeting flocked together. The sun pressing its murk from outside. Spring going the color of steel.

At the crest of the stairs, you hear your two aunts. Karen. Lynn. Karen's husband runs the dealership, takes advantage of his brother-in-law. Karen and your mother do not talk. They talk now. Their talk brothering the kitchen.

The voices bear the sheen of linoleum, and from this echo, you know they are in the kitchen. Four cups of coffee ringing the table—these women, these aunts, mothers, and sisters, drinking with faces veiled in steam. Drone. The standing of Heather, her silent coming to your side. Your careful sit into the chair. They look, stop looking, look forever, stop.

Your mother brings you orange tea. You hate coffee. She knows that. She brings you tea in a white cup etched with hummingbirds. Adds the half-teaspoon of sugar for you, stirs for you, stares for you, into the swirling amber. Your face in the softness of her chest. You cry so briefly.

She talks of the funeral, the arrangements, tomorrow already, not pleased that you have come downstairs to hear this. Not pleased. You are so curious about the details. The coffin, the speeches, the drive to *the cemetery, the looking out the window at a season developing. She asks if you want to stay, to hear the details, and you say you do. The details, though, are at the playground, sifting paper from the woodchips. The lie of something so overwhelmingly true. Like a glass overfilled, this truth spills its sides, makes a mess, stains the tablecloth. In this, your mother can not continue. Aunt Lynn's husband, Joe, completes the arrangements. The pathetic chandelier husbands your mother's hair. Dyed black.*

That night, at Aunt Lynn's house, different beds. Your mother will not stay at home. You sleep with her in her arms. In her arms, you don't sleep with her. You roll your fist into your mother's, feel the chill of her ring. She clasps you as if in a claw. She knows. You are your father's daughter.

Of course. Rain. Of course, hot mugs, drinks, and toast before leaving. The brown toast. The piano under the dust. The Earth knowing what we do, and don't. Of course, black clothes, but you have no dresses in that color. Instead, the beige dress your parents bought you for your last birthday. This matters. Your first funeral. Your first funeral is your father's. How to behave? What are people going to say? Shuffles of cloth, long empty tables with fold-out legs. Behind long empty tables with fold-out legs, the broken swish of so many black sleeves. How parents is a word that no longer belongs to you.

Strange how we lose things. Strange how so many things lose us. We are unfound, here. Unfound in this car, your aunt's, the hands on the steering wheel, your aunt's. Your mother in the passenger seat, your sister beside you in the back. Separately lost. The armrest between you is unbreachable and maroon. The rain scolding the window. The windshield wipers allowing you to see clearly, if only for a second. The clouds full, distended, almost black. So low, slipped from the hands of the sky. The chapel coming at the corner. The heart struggling to remember its only word.

In the chapel, the faces. The people to face. The walls creamed with paint, the living flowers plump with their water. Curtains hiding so many eulogies in their folds. Your mother is with you. Heather is with you. This, you tell yourself. The friends and family, obligatory, predatory, warm.

The funeral director, long fingers, complexion of popsicle sticks, some juvenile arts and crafts project, calls your mother into his study. His voice held together with paste. You cling to Heather, the black cotton of her arm, finding a kind of fire there. The kind that burns out. The friends and family stare as if you're in cages, the charity of looking, the charity of looking away.

Heather, six years above you, touches your shoulder. You are girls. Walking through a crowd and nodding. This chorus of sorrys, almost funny. Without anchor, nothing but a collection of sounds, never gelling into song. In just a few years, Heather will disappear into cancer, then disappear for good. You will never show anyone your writing, before you stop writing altogether, losing yourself in teaching English to seventh graders—Animal Farm, Jane Eyre, A Separate Peace.

You look nowhere, but at the casket.

Brown, cold. His body inside, lidded, so impossible. It must be empty. It looks empty. Wonder if he is comfortable. Wonder if he is warm enough. Answers surely inscribed inside. Written in a dying ink.

The rabbi, beardless, approaches the podium and begins his eulogy. The microphone wobbling on its skinny stand. His cheeks are so red, like a child's. Pock-marked. You've known him for a long time, remember him with a full brown beard that covered the top of his neck. You like him very much, but wish him away. Into the pillars and candles. Into their smoke. If he wasn't talking, you wouldn't have to listen.

Such a good man, he says, his throat wealthy, bursting with fat. Such a good man, and you picture him with the jack, the tickets to the circus where he bought you peanuts in a paper bag, your first lion. The acrobats so lovely in their leotards with names that came from so far away. Names with Ys and Zs, and hands that didn't fail them, even when upside-down.

A good man, he says, hair going gray at the tips, something your *father's hair will not receive the chance to do. Flowing black robe, this ringmaster of soft, kind words, the tragedy of announcement. A short speech. Mentioning the entire family. Speaking your name. In this, strength and its shedding, a new exposed skin. He knows, the rabbi. How much love it takes. Commerce. How much he was loved. Will be missed. An ad for a used piano. Someone circling with a red pen. We are light. How the rest of your life will be obvious.*

Sixteen

A SWEATY WAKING in the Cimarron. Johanna's eyes open. Coming to temperature, and decision. In her neck, all the sweet-sour sleep smells responsible, in waking, for movement. In the morning, she does not report for massage duty. I do not walk to the fields. For breakfast, cantaloupe and soy milk. Even Alex, Emily, and Antonio are winding down. Opening a carton. Removing a peel. We do what we've been thinking about doing. Johanna and I have to see things in Chicago through to their end. Then restart. Open a carton. Remove a peel.

When we tell Charlie that we are leaving to be with the family through the final few stages of . . . *healing?* . . . he says, "Bout time, brother," as if he were waiting for us to come to this. As if Vietnam and death and booze have made such things obvious to him, but allowed him the patience not to give us any shit about it. He hugs me into his beard, stinking of pot. Even before he lets me go, his hug, the smell of him, the pressure of his fingertips on my back, becomes memory, however faulty. He is nodding. He readjusts his shirt collar and is nodding. He doesn't say another *brother*.

Lance, too, is unsurprised. "Shiiit," he croons, "I'll miss your presence," then catches himself. "Presences."

He pulls at Ruby's fingers, cracking one of them. Somewhere, miles away, so many people wait for him to read to them. Bob and the German Shepherd are arm wrestling under the dining tent to see who gets the last piece of cantaloupe. It's a piece that was cut close to the rind and still has that sheen of white and green rimming the orange flesh. Bob hums, breathlessly, "Magic Carpet Ride." This is a lie, but imagine if it weren't. While they struggle, Charlie palms the melon slice, slides it down his own throat. On the foreheads of Bob and the Shepherd, more sweat. In their eyes, endless *what the fucks?!*

Lady Wanda kisses Johanna on the lips. A long kiss, her wonderful arm wrapped around my wife's neck, Johanna's blonde hair becoming the necklace at Lady Wanda's middle. Lady Wanda hands me a manila envelope of rubber-banded cash.

"The Meaning of Work," I say.

Lady Wanda laughs a throaty "Go fuck yourself, honey," then licks my face, my beard, against the grain. Yes. She really does this.

"Norman'll take ya to your car."

Portions of the crew return to the crops. Leaving their signatures behind—their breakfast plates in the trash, their tents in the Residents' Camp. Ours this morning deflated like a balloon. Left an octagon of dead grass in its place. Our marker. Our graffiti. It's like summer camp or senior year. I want to write *Have a Good Summer* on the backs of everyone's weed-stained hands. In fact, a few crew members sign their names to our xeroxed copy of Lady Wanda's manifesto—Norman: "with affection"; the German Shepherd, strangely equipped with a tin of black ink, leaves his thumbprint.

From Alex, Emily, Antonio, and Robbi, only salutes. Simultaneous salutes as if they had practiced this like yoga, rehearsed illicitly in the walk-in fridge, in between French kisses and veggie burgers. A quadruple salutation.

The air is cool and cooling. In it, the redwoods creak, Hector somewhere perched in them, listening to Dr. Judy on his radio chastising yet another unfaithful man, eating his thin sandwich. Certainly he must be watching us depart, the goodbyes a surprise, like his lunch, easily swallowed. Crazy Jeff is nowhere to be found. Nobody knows where he's gone. Johanna and I are a little worried.

Norman drives us to the spur road parking lot in the sporty green and white golf cart. His beard whipping. His "End of the Trail" belt buckle reflecting the grayness of the sky. In it, swirling above us, Gloria is surely healthy enough to drive, my Grandpa Max selling her a used car. We become what we used to be. Salesmen. Women. Daughters. Sons.

Johanna holds my hand the entire way. We pass through two of the four gates that bar entrance to Weckman, and spin left up the spur road toward the grassy lot in which, a lifetime ago, we ditched our car. The Kia Spectra. Red. Illinois plates. The cool metal. The stuff, nearly, of the womb. Collecting condensation and stench. Norman is telling us one last story. Johanna and I are listening.

"Dude, while I was in line at the drugstore, this homeless guy who looks just like me walks in, steals something, and runs out. The girl at the register—pretty young, short red hair—is a little alarmed. 'What did he take?' she asks me. 'I don't know,' I say. 'I think it was a candy bar.' 'Okay,' she says. 'I'll let him go then.' 'I think that's a good thing,' I say. 'A good idea.' Then, we start talking, and I'm wearing what I'm wearing now."

(Black nightgown, black cowboy boots, jeans, a necklace of crystals and Tibetan amulets.)

"And she asks me about my crystals, and I tell her all the spiritual shit, dude. So she looks at me, right in the eyes, and says, just like this, 'Old man, I like your style,' as she drops . . . my Preparation H . . . into the paper bag."

Johanna smiles like she's going to cry. I want to laugh. I really do. I'm going to miss these people. The perspective. The golf carts. The softness of the rugs they pull out from under us. Their non-suburban-Chicago-ness.

"Mm-haaa-aaa!" Norman bellows and deposits us, dazed and lip-biting, into the parking lot.

His hug is bread warm, his chest and beard smelling of allspice. When he hugs Johanna, she whispers something in his ear and he does not laugh. He walks backward, remounts the cart. Starts it. Doesn't pause.

"Love you guys!" he shouts. "Catch ya!"

He spins the wheel and floors his contraption, his spirit animal, back toward Weckman proper. Johanna and I face one another, find our Kia in a sea of VW Buses, 1980s Cadillacs, two rusty convertibles. In the grass, in the trees, the cicadas clack their castanets. The whispering of thousands of instruments, the beating of so many foreign hearts. Not a single other human thing.

I sigh. Johanna corrects this, and kisses me. Here, in this field, we don't have to control ourselves. There is nothing to control. The air is cool and the grass already wears tomorrow's dew. We look around out of habit, knowing we don't have to. Our dirty shoes come off first—the hardest of the garments. Then our shirts. Johanna's is thin and blue. After all these years, she still has to help me with the buttons.

DID I HAVE SEX with my wife on the cool hood of that Kia, in that isolated lot? Yes. Yes. Yes I did. And it was everything I hoped sex with my wife and a Kia Spectra hood would be—hot and metal and revved-up and transmittive and explosive and gear-shifting and gas guzzling and accelerating and alternating and . . . Yes. I know. That's enough. We started at Point A, arrived at Point B, and this time, B is better.

When we've finished, and unlock the doors, the car is revolting. Filthy, musty, not a single window left cracked.

"I hope it starts," Johanna says.

I am grateful for her voice, the Swedish in it, so out of place in the screams of California cicadas, this commingling of species. The doors suck open, the floorboards littered with the old styrofoam to-go boxes, poppyseeds, breadcrumbs gathered on our road trip out here. The things we so long ago consumed. The places we ate, and filled up with gasoline. Johanna folds herself into the passenger seat and reaches for the radio before I turn on the car. She kicks at an empty plastic bottle of strawberry milk. The Kia sags with our weight and I expect it to creak. The key. The ignition. The car starts right up.

DRIVING AT DUSK, the satellites come out over the desert. The sky through the windshield is a painful blue, the moon like some lewd headlamp parting the knots of creosote. Somewhere, so many tired people are harvesting marijuana. Johanna has had her hand on my leg for over an hour, the sweat cooling between our skins. We are driving toward.

We don't say much, listen to the radio, some jazz followed by talk, some former gang member talking about how poetry saved his life, how he remembered his first convenience store that wasn't equipped with bulletproof glass. Perspective.

Around the car, this whip of red mineral sands, the moon whiting the desert like a page. Raw. Full of unseen skulls. The salt of the primordial ocean. We drive. Few cars. Hands cramped on the wheel. Johanna watching her own face in the side-view mirror. I want to see what she sees. In our chests, the bracing for Chicago, for good news, bad news, reheated food and loud breakfasts. The ham at the end of the desert. The mother there.

"The sky gets so dark out here," I say to Johanna, and want to continue with talking about something, anything, the desert around us, steeped in its dry allegiances, birds dropping dead into the centers of flowering cacti.

"Good for stars," Johanna says, and it's night.

Soon, Johanna is snoring, and it's amazing to hear this in something other than a tent. It's night, and we drive through it, fleeing the edge of America, by the green digitals of the clock—driving fast and east, still in the final hold of coastal things, this time zone so assertive and decidedly Pacific. Where we're headed, it's later.

I put my hand on Johanna's thigh, and through the windshield, the insects sacrificed to our speed, I feel some sort of lifetime stretch out before us. In its infinity, its road-acoustics and sweet nighttime desert smells, I feel strong and stupid, confused, doomed, excited, broken with love, and, as long as I keep driving, finally reliable.

ALSO BY MATTHEW GAVIN FRANK

Barolo
(University of Nebraska Press, 2010)

Warranty in Zulu
(Barrow Street Press, 2010)

Sagittarius Agitprop
(Black Lawrence Press/Dzanc Books, 2009)